Exercise Prescription for Fitness

Exercise Prescription
for Fitness

J. GAVIN REID / JOHN M. THOMSON
Queen's University, Kingston, Canada

PRENTICE-HALL, INC., Englewood Cliffs, New Jersey 07632

Library of Congress Cataloging in Publication Data

REID, J. GAVIN.
  Exercise prescription for fitness.

  Includes bibliographies and index.
  1. Exercise.   2. Exercise—Physiological aspects.
  3. Physical fitness.   I. Thomson, John M. (date)
II. Title.
GV481.R44 1985   613.7'1   84-18084
ISBN 0-13-294638-6

GV
481
.R44
1985

Editorial/production supervision and
  interior design: *Hilda Tauber; Fred Bernardi*
Cover design: *Lundgren Graphics, Ltd.*
Cover logo courtesy *Track and Field Journal,*
  Canadian Track and Field Association, Sports Canada
Manufacturing buyer: *Harry P. Baisley*

Printed in the United States of America

10 9 8 7 6 5 4 3 2 1

ISBN 0-13-294638-6   01

PRENTICE-HALL INTERNATIONAL, INC., *London*
PRENTICE-HALL OF AUSTRALIA PTY. LIMITED, *Sydney*
EDITORA PRENTICE-HALL DO BRASIL, LTDA., *Rio de Janeiro*
PRENTICE-HALL CANADA INC., *Toronto*
PRENTICE-HALL HISPANOAMERICANA, S.A., *Mexico*
PRENTICE-HALL OF INDIA PRIVATE LIMITED, *New Delhi*
PRENTICE-HALL OF JAPAN, INC., *Tokyo*
PRENTICE-HALL OF SOUTHEAST ASIA PTE. LTD., *Singapore*
WHITEHALL BOOKS LIMITED, *Wellington, New Zealand*

To our wives, Patricia and Anne

Contents

3 Skeletal and Muscular Function   *12*

4 Human Posture: Structure and Dynamics   *26*

PART III: PHYSIOLOGICAL CONSIDERATIONS

5 Muscle Energetics   *44*

6 The Physiological Systems: Support for Muscle Activity   62

PART IV: PERSONALIZED EXERCISE PRESCRIPTION

7 Personal Fitness Evaluation   105

8 Personal Fitness Prescription   152

9 Alternative Activity Prescriptions *198*

Preface

During the last fifteen years, North America has experienced a fitness boom. The initial jogging craze of the 1970s has expanded rapidly into a myriad of fitness-related areas and activities. In the 1980s a wide variety of exercise and movement programs are being offered at colleges, YM/YWCAs, fitness and recreational centers, industrial complexes, downtown businesses, in the suburbs, and even in the basement of homes. The number of fitness specialists also has increased rapidly to meet these growing needs. Although the number of publications in the area of fitness has also proliferated in recent years, most of them fall into two opposing categories. At one extreme are the books and magazines offering plenty of information on how to perform specific exercises and activities, but little or no scientific explanations. At the opposite extreme are the texts conveying detailed scientific information on fitness, but very little by way of practical applications.

This text meets the growing need to bridge these two extremes. In Parts I and II we give the reader a basic understanding of the concepts and scientific facts relating to health and fitness; in Parts III and IV we provide specific practical information that can be applied directly. The book also includes a battery of fitness tests that are thorough yet easily performed, a simple percentile scoring system for each test, and detailed instructions for evaluating (or for periodically reevaluating) one's fitness. Based upon the test scores obtained and their evaluation, the reader can formulate an individualized exercise program—his or her *personal prescription* for fitness.

Designed primarily for undergraduate college students, this text may also be useful for graduate students studying physical fitness, for fitness professionals working in the field, and for individual health enthusiasts who are concerned with and wish to learn more about their personal fitness. The central objectives of this text are to provide the student or practitioner with a sound knowledge of the anatomical and physiological bases of fitness exercise, plus the self-testing fitness profile and in-depth analyses to complement this understanding. The entire process—shown as a model in Chapter 1—has been designed so that readers can make intelligent decisions regarding their personal fitness: the type of exercise program (or programs) to embark upon, why certain choices are best suited for them, specific risks to avoid when exercising, and so on.

In writing this text we especially wanted to give our readers information of *practical* value. One major emphasis, for example, is on correct posture and how to achieve it—a topic that is seldom covered in texts dealing specifically with personal fitness. We also discuss several myths and controversies, such as spot weight reduction, and we try to answer questions pertaining to lifestyle and the role that fitness can play in it. In the appendixes we provide reference materials on functional human anatomy, metric conversion tables, and the general fitness guidelines recommended by the American College of Sports Medicine.

ACKNOWLEDGMENTS

The authors are indebted to a number of friends and associates for their timely assistance and enthusiastic support.

We are grateful to Donald Macintosh, our mentor, friend, and colleague, for his guidance and inspiration over the years. To our typists, Betty Schieck and Dorothy Daley we extend our appreciation for their many hours of labor. Our sincere thanks go to Meredith Galbraith, who prepared most of the line drawings for the book, and to the students who posed as subjects for the photographs.

Last but by no means least, we express our appreciation to our wives, Patricia Reid and Anne Thomson, who gave their support, encouragement, and much-needed assistance throughout the preparation of the manuscript.

J. GAVIN REID

JOHN M. THOMSON

Exercise Prescription for Fitness

1

Model for Exercise Prescription

WHAT IS FITNESS AND EXERCISE PRESCRIPTION?

Fitness! What is it really? At times, no field appears as confusing and misunderstood as that of physical fitness and sports training. Few disciplines have perpetuated as many myths, utilized as much jargon, and created such a plethora of "experts," yet there may be no discipline as clearly understood and as practical when applied. The expression *being in shape,* when used in reference to a person's preparedness for physical activity, has very little meaning and can actually prove quite misleading. A person who is in shape is physically prepared for only a limited range of athletic endeavors. A *universal* preparedness—that is, a readiness for all physical activities and sports—is highly improbable because of the limits of the biomechanical and physiological capabilities that any individual can possess, even with intense training. Consider the athletic spectrum: the sprinter, the Olympic weight lifter, the elite marathon runner, and the everyday jogger. All may well be in shape, but only for their specific athletic pursuit. The competitive athlete is tuned for a specific sports event: the marathoner, for example, cannot compete successfully at highly competitive levels in either sprinting or weight lifting, and the jogger, following a reasonable and proper exercise prescription, will be in shape for jogging. But although most athletes are in shape primarily for their chosen physical activity, they may have different reasons for wanting to be in shape: highly competitive athletes may wish to place themselves among the elite in their sport, whereas the jogger may exercise for enjoyment, to improve cardiovascular health, to promote a feeling of well-being, or to have social interaction with friends.

There are so many fitness recipes! A few are useful, many are not, and unfortunately some can prove injurious to the participant. Millions of people believe that spot reduction of subcutaneous fat in specific locales is possible, and gadgets, belts, pills, and exercises that perpetuate this myth are still merchandised. Diet books, some with suspect scientific information, still become best sellers. Some people sit in steam baths, lose a small amount of their body water through sweating, then believe they have burned up calories in the heat; others try to roll and pound their body fat away. Every day across North America people lie on their living-room floor with their ankles and wrists affixed to a pulley system, flailing their limbs against gravity and the resistance of the pulley. There are even people who bob up and down on a flexible chaise longue, probably doing irreparable damage to their spine and lower back in the name of fitness. By far the majority of people interested in fitness are found daily in front of their TV sets lying, sitting, stretching, jumping, tumbling, or mumbling as they follow the gyrations of their favorite exercise guru. Hippocrates claimed that all parts of the body that have a function become healthy, well developed, and slow to age if exercised; if they are not exercised, they become liable to disease, defective in growth, and quick to age[1]. Some two thousand years later, this claim cannot be refuted on scientific grounds and is still regarded as the basis for the prescription of exercise for physical fitness.

This book is concerned with fitness—what it is and how it can be maintained or modified. It emphasizes the components of fitness and how each affects one's health. Physical fitness is more than just a clean bill of health following a routine medical examination. It is, rather, a level of bodily efficiency encompassing two major areas. The first is *anatomy*, in particular the musculoskeletal system—bones, joints, and muscles, and their interrelation in posture and in the basic skills of locomotion, such as walking, running, and lifting. The second major area is *physiology*, especially the functional excellence of the respiratory and circulatory system; the muscles; anthropometric considerations, such as low body fat; overall body composition and aesthetic considerations; basic motor fitness (flexibility, strength, and so forth); and nutrition. There are many other physiological considerations as well, some of medical concern, such as the sense organs, endocrinology, the digestive system, and the internal organs. Figure 1.1 shows the continuum of health and fitness.

Anatomical Considerations

Knowledge of the effects of various levels of intensity of exercise or lack of it on the growth and development of bone and joints is vitally important to anyone prescribing exercises for fitness. Exercises incorrectly performed may be hazardous to the healthy growth and condition of the skeletal system not only

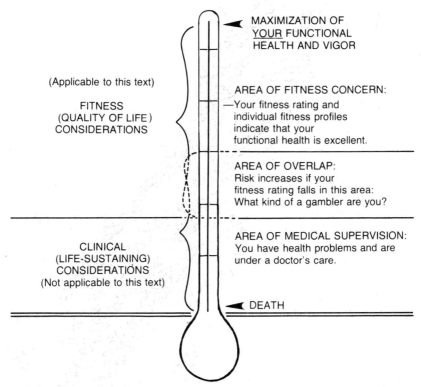

MAXIMIZATION OF
YOUR FUNCTIONAL
HEALTH AND VIGOR

(Applicable to this text)

FITNESS
(QUALITY OF LIFE)
CONSIDERATIONS

AREA OF FITNESS CONCERN:
—Your fitness rating and
individual fitness profiles
indicate that your
functional health is excellent.

AREA OF OVERLAP:
Risk increases if your
fitness rating falls in this area:
What kind of a gambler are you?

CLINICAL
(LIFE-SUSTAINING)
CONSIDERATIONS
(Not applicable to this text)

AREA OF MEDICAL SUPERVISION:
You have health problems and are
under a doctor's care.

DEATH

FIGURE 1.1 The health and fitness continuum. Through exercise prescription each individual chooses a position on the continuum. If you don't aim high enough for your fitness capacity, you may risk dropping into the area requiring medical attention in the future.

of the growing child, but also of the conditioned athlete, the sedentary person who has not exercised for a number of years, and the aged. It is also very important for anyone concerned with the prescription of exercise to be aware of the movement capability and limitation of the bones and joints. To detect defects and correctly prescribe exercises for these conditions, one must have a clear understanding of what is normal structure and normal movement.

Knowledge of the structure and function of muscle is another important anatomical consideration. How is it possible to fix or improve a system or machine if one is not familiar with how it is constructed and how it works? One needs to become aware not only of the role of the individual muscles in simple motion, but also of the complexity of the relationship between muscles and skeletal parts during movement. Muscles do not act independently; there is a constant interplay between muscles or between groups of muscles during even the simplest of movements. This book emphasizes knowledge of muscles because of its importance to the exercise prescriptionist, who may be concerned with the rehabilitation of an injury, the development of specific muscles for a specific task, or the design of an exercise program for the harmonious development of the muscles of the body.

One of the most neglected areas in physical-fitness and physical-education programs is that of posture. The correct alignment of the bones and joints, not only in static positions such as standing and sitting but also during the dynamic movements of locomotion, is of great importance to one's health and to efficient movement. Specific exercises can be prescribed that improve posture by strengthening muscle and increasing the extensibility of muscle, ligaments, and tendons, thereby realigning the skeletal parts.

Physiological Considerations

The basis of all physical exercise is muscular contraction. Thus an important physiological consideration must be the sources of energy available for muscular activity. The energy for exercise, unlike the combustion engine of a car, can come from more than one source. Which intramuscular source(s) should be utilized, and to what degree, must be well understood before one embarks upon any type of fitness program, for the intensity and type of exercise undertaken have a significant effect upon the functioning of the entire body.

The synchronous elevation of a number of physiological systems—the respiratory and cardiovascular systems in particular—is a very important consideration. There are healthful and proper ways to stress these systems. On the other hand, inappropriate physical activities can impose inordinate stresses and strains upon the body. Thus the intensity, duration, and type of exercise for one person can prove to be of little value or even harmful (too stressful) for another.

Another important physiological consideration is diet and nutrition. A great deal has been written about diet and the nutritional requirements imposed on the body by exercise. However, much of this information has abetted the myth that exercise *alone* is a good method of mass (weight) control.* Criteria for determining one's amount of body fat are specified in Chapter 6, and body composition is discussed in detail. Specific motor-fitness capabilities, flexibility and strength, are also quantified.

The emphasis of this book is on integration—integration of the anatomical and physiological aspects of fitness, and integration of information and knowledge about fitness into a personalized fitness prescription. This book provides for individual analysis so that a self-testing fitness profile can be developed; specific fitness prescriptions are recommended that not only tell the individual what to do, but also explain the anatomical and physiological bases of the prescription as well as specific exercises and risks to be avoided. Finally, this book clearly differentiates between personal fitness and training for specific sports, for most people believe they are one and the same thing; nothing could be further from the truth.

---

* Note the definitions of body mass and body weight in the glossary.

FIGURE 1.2 MODEL FOR PERSONAL FITNESS PRESCRIPTION

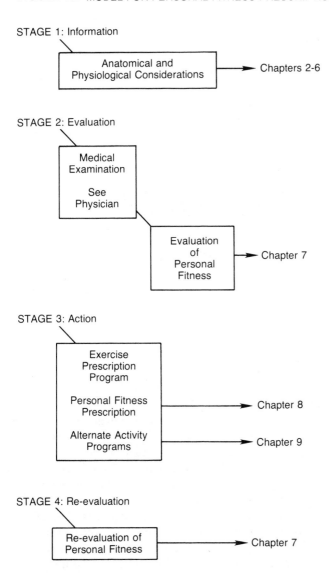

STAGE 1: Information

> Anatomical and Physiological Considerations → Chapters 2-6

STAGE 2: Evaluation

> Medical Examination
>
> See Physician
>
> Evaluation of Personal Fitness → Chapter 7

STAGE 3: Action

> Exercise Prescription Program
>
> Personal Fitness Prescription → Chapter 8
>
> Alternate Activity Programs → Chapter 9

STAGE 4: Re-evaluation

> Re-evaluation of Personal Fitness → Chapter 7

Figure 1.2 is the model we will use in this book for personal fitness prescription.

REFERENCES

1. *Hippocrates,* trans. E. T. Withington (New York: Putnam's, 1927), pp. 339, 341.

2

Basic Terminology

INTRODUCTION

Anatomy is the science of the structure of the human body and the relation of its parts. It is based largely on dissection, from which it obtains its name[1]. The study of the structure of the human body is paramount to an understanding of its function: it is necessary for a working understanding of the methods used in the rehabilitation of an injured or malfunctioning part of the body, in the maintenance of a healthy and well-functioning body, and in the improvement of the capacity of the human body to perform physical tasks. It is important to know how the human body creates and responds to internal and external stresses that influence its structure and function. An understanding of fitness and how exercise affects it requires a basic knowledge of both the anatomy (structure) and physiology (function) of the body. The latter will be discussed in Part III.

The purpose of this chapter is to present the basic concepts of anatomy necessary for exercise prescription for fitness. This information is an absolute minimum, and we strongly advise you to take additional courses in human anatomy and physiology in order to gain a more thorough understanding of the functioning of the body.

To accurately explain an exercise to someone, it is necessary to have a thorough knowledge of the names of skeletal parts and major muscles and a familiarity with the basic terminology used for describing human motion. Use Appendix A for a review of the parts of the skeleton and the muscles of the body and their locations, origins, insertions, and actions. In this chapter we discuss the basic concepts of standing position, planes and axes, directional terms, and fundamental movements.

ANATOMICAL POSITION

The standing position is commonly regarded as an upright stance in which the feet are close together, the head is held comfortably erect, and the arms hang relaxed at the sides. This is indeed the starting position for many exercises, but in order to correctly describe the movements that occur at the various joints of the body, it is necessary to visualize the body in a standardized reference position that is slightly different from the one just described. This position, which is used by anatomists, physical educators, and other exercise specialists, is called the anatomical position. Figure 2.1 illustrates this position; note the erect posture of the trunk and neck, the supinated forearms, and the straight legs with the feet together.

PLANES AND AXES

The three cardinal orientation planes that correspond to the three dimensions of space are used to describe positions and movements of the body (Figure 2.2). The *sagittal plane* is a vertical plane that divides the body into left and right parts. The *frontal plane* divides the body into anterior (front) and posterior (back) parts. The *transverse plane* is a horizontal plane that divides the body into superior (top) and inferior (bottom) parts. When a plane divides the body into two equal masses it is called a midplane; therefore, the center of mass of the body is the point where the midsagittal, midfrontal, and midtransverse planes intersect.

A body part that moves parallel to one of these planes is said to move in the sagittal, frontal, or transverse plane. Describing movement in terms of these planes is very useful in explaining exercises. Remember that the body planes remain the same regardless of the orientation of the body to the earth: when describing a movement performed in any of the planes, refer back to the anatomical position for a reference point.

Corresponding to the three planes of motion are three anatomical axes, each associated with one plane of motion and perpendicular to that plane:

1. The *transverse axis* passes through the body from side to side; associated with the *sagittal plane*.

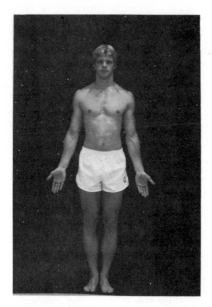

FIGURE 2.1
The anatomical position.

2. The *anteroposterior axis* passes through the body from anterior to posterior; associated with the *frontal plane.*
3. The *longitudinal axis* passes through the body from superior to inferior; associated with the *transverse plane*[2].

DIRECTIONAL TERMS

It is important to be aware of the spatial terms that are used in discussing the human body. These are defined in Table 2.1. If we look at Figure 2.1 we can see that: the head is superior to the trunk while the feet are inferior to the trunk; the fingers are distal to the elbows while the shoulders are proximal to the elbows; the small finger is the most medial of the digits of the hand and the thumb is the most lateral. Figure 2.1 presents the anterior view of the body; the posterior surface is not visible.

As with planes of the body, these terms are referenced to the anatomical position and not to the earth. Even if the subject of Figure 2.1 were to be standing on his head, the terms would be the same. For example, the head is always superior to the trunk. If our subject in Figure 2.1 had the palms of his hands facing away from us, the thumbs would still be the most lateral digits and the visible surface of the hands (the backs of the hands) would still be their posterior surface. The only difference would be that the forearms had been pronated.

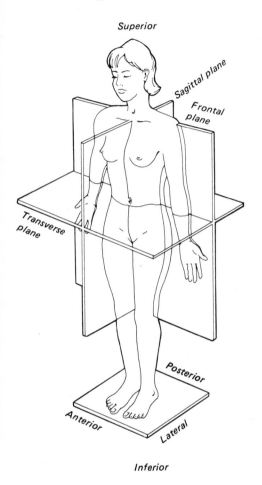

Superior

Sagittal plane

Frontal plane

Transverse plane

Posterior

Anterior

Lateral

Inferior

FIGURE 2.2
Orientation planes, anatomical position. *Source*: Adapted from James G. Hay and J. Gavin Reid, *The Anatomical and Mechanical Bases of Human Motion* © 1982, p. 10. Reprinted by permission of Prentice-Hall, Inc., Englewood Cliffs, N.J.

FUNDAMENTAL MOVEMENTS

Movements in the Sagittal Plane

All movements in the sagittal plane occur around transverse axes. The possible movements in this plane include flexion, extension, hyperextension, plantar flexion, and dorsi flexion. In the anatomical position, all joints are regarded as being in full extension. If the angle between joining bones is decreasing in the sagittal plane, *flexion* is occurring at the joint; the opposite action, which results in an increasing angle, is *extension*. If a joint moves beyond the fully extended position, *hyperextension* results. Plantar flexion and dorsi flexion are terms for describing movement in the sagittal plane at the ankle joint. *Plantar*

TABLE 2.1 Positional/Directional Terms (referenced to the anatomical position)

Superior	At or toward plane of the head
Inferior	At or toward plane of the feet
Distal	At or toward the hands or feet
Proximal	Closer to the body (trunk)
Medial	Toward the midline of body
Lateral	Away from the midline of body
Anterior	Located in front of the midfrontal plane
Posterior	Located behind the midfrontal plane

flexion raises the standing body onto its toes; *dorsi flexion* is the movement of the anterior (top) surface of the foot towards the tibia (shin). These five movements, and those in the frontal and transverse planes, are summarized in Table 2.2.

Movements in the Frontal Plane

Movements that occur in the frontal plane are abduction, adduction, elevation, depression, and lateral bending. Movement of a body part away from the midline of the body in the frontal plane (that is, on the anteroposterior axis) is called *abduction*. An example is the lateral raising of the arm from the side

TABLE 2.2 Fundamental Movements

PLANE	AXIS	ACTION	DEFINITION
Sagittal	Transverse	Flexion	Decreasing the angle between two bones
		Extension	Increasing the angle between two bones
		Hyperextension	Overextension (moving beyond full extension)
		Plantar Flexion	Moving the sole of the foot downward
		Dorsi Flexion	Moving the top of the foot upward
Frontal	Anteroposterior	Abduction	Moving away from middle of body or part
		Adduction	Moving toward midline of body or part
		Elevation	Moving to superior position
		Depression	Moving to inferior position
		Lateral Bending	Bending spinal column to side
Transverse	Longitudinal	Rotation	Turning about the vertical axis of the bone
		Supination	Rotating forearm laterally
		Pronation	Rotating forearm medially

of the body. The returning of the arm towards the body is an example of *adduction*. When the arm is abducted to shoulder level and is then moved toward the midline of the body in the transverse plane, the action is called horizontal adduction. Movement back to the abducted position is called horizontal abduction[3]. *Elevation* and *depression* are the respective terms for the raising and lowering of the shoulder girdle, as in shrugging the shoulders. The final movement in the frontal plane is *lateral bending* (to the left or right) of the spinal column or regions of it.

Movements in the Transverse Plane

Movements of *rotation* in the transverse plane occur around longitudinal axes. The direction of movement is referenced to the anterior surface of the trunk or of the limb in question. For example, when we say that rotation of the trunk is either to the left or right, we mean that the anterior surface of the trunk rotates in one of these directions. Rotation of a limb is described as inward or medial when the anterior surface moves toward the midline of the body, and outward or lateral when the anterior surface moves away from the midline. Supination and pronation are movements of the forearm. In the anatomical position, the forearms are in a position of *supination*—that is, a position of outward or lateral rotation. Inward or medial rotation of the forearms resulting in the palms of the hands facing the body is called *pronation*.

REFERENCES

1. *Dorland's Illustrated Medical Dictionary*, 24th ed. (Philadelphia: Saunders, 1965), p. 79.
2. James G. Hay and J. Gavin Reid, *The Anatomical and Mechanical Bases of Human Motion* (Englewood Cliffs, N.J.: Prentice-Hall, 1982), p. 11.
3. Ibid., p. 13.

3

Skeletal and Muscular Function

INTRODUCTION

The human skeleton contains between 206 and 210 bones. Nearly all of these bones articulate at joints, most of which are supported by ligaments, cartilages, fasciae, and tendons. The skeletal system provides firm support for the attachments of approximately 500 muscles and numerous ligaments and fasciae, and is thus the basis of leverage and movement. (Refer to Appendix A for a review of the bones and muscles of the body.) Furthermore, the skeleton protects many of the vital organs of the body. For example, the lungs and heart are contained in the thoracic cage, and the brain is encased in the cranium. The skeletal muscles constitute almost 40 percent of the total body mass and contain thousands of multinucleate single-cell muscle fibers that are stimulated by an enormous network of nerve tissue[1].

The purpose of this chapter is to provide a basic understanding of the effects of exercise on the development of the skeletal system, the properties of connective tissues in joint mobility, and the effects of exercise on the development of range of motion at joints. In addition, we offer a brief explanation of the muscular system, discussing such topics as muscle structure, types of muscular contraction, the effects of exercise on the development of muscular strength and endurance, and the various muscle groups.

THE SKELETAL SYSTEM

Structure of Bone

Approximately two-thirds of the mass of bone consists of inorganic matter, mainly calcium phosphate and calcium carbonate. The remaining one-third is organic and composed largely of collagen fibers. The ratio of inorganic to organic matter varies with age. The bones of the very young contain a high percentage of organic matter, which makes them soft and flexible; those of the aged lose much of their organic matter and become much more brittle.

There are two types of bony substance: *compact tissue* (the hard outer layer of bone) and *cancellous tissue* (the spongelike tissue found within the outer case of compact bone). Compact bone is able to withstand great *stress* (the load per unit area that develops in response to a force that is applied from without). Cancellous tissue is lighter than compact tissue but is strong and resistant to *strain* (the deformation—lengthening or shortening—within a structure while it is being loaded). Together they provide an effective structure for withstanding the stresses and strains of everyday activities, including exercise.

Growth and Development of Bone

Bones develop from the embryonic connective tissue called *mesenchyme* into either *intramembranous* or *endochondral* bones. The former are the flat bones of the body, such as those of the skull. The latter become the long bones, in which *ossification* (the process of bone formation) first occurs at the center of a cartilage model of the bone and spreads toward the ends. Near the ends of long bones are growth zones called *epiphyseal disks*; it is here that the shaft of a bone lengthens. There are two types of epiphyses—traction and pressure[2]. *Traction epiphyses* are found at the bony origins and insertions of many muscles of the body. In Figure 3.1 a traction epiphysis is shown at the proximal end of the ulna, to which the triceps muscle is attached; also shown is a pressure epiphysis on the radius.

The closure of the center of ossification in a bone takes place from about six to twenty years of age. During these years, and particularly at the prepubescent and pubescent stages of growth, the epiphyseal disks are susceptible to injury due to a traumatic impact or repeated impacts of high intensity and may close prematurely. This will result in stunted growth of the bone. For this reason, among others, selection of exercises and physical activities should be done with care and good protective equipment should be used in high-impact activities. On the other hand, the importance of exercises for the healthy development of bone cannot be overemphasized. Exercises that provide moderate stress and strain to bones stimulate healthy growth. Bone is living material and adapts to

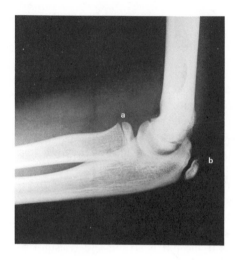

FIGURE 3.1
(a) Pressure epiphysis on radius; (b) traction epiphysis at proximal end of ulna. *Source*: James G. Hay and J. Gavin Reid, *The Anatomical and Mechanical Bases of Human Motion* © 1982, p. 21. Reprinted by permission of Prentice-Hall, Inc., Englewood Cliffs, N.J.

stimuli that are not too traumatic. Inactivity, such as prolonged bed rest or casting (following the breaking of a bone), results in a rapid loss of mineral substances in bones and therefore a reduction in their strength.

Movement of Articulating Bone: Joint Flexibility

Many of the factors governing movement have been scientifically studied. The range through which joints move is one of the most important of these factors. Without flexibility movement is impossible; with limited flexibility movement and other human functions are inefficient.

The study of flexibility has produced controversy. For one thing, the change in angle at a joint has been variously termed *mobilization, freedom to move, range of motion in joints,* and, most commonly, *flexibility.* Whether the flexibility characteristics of the body are general or specific to the individual is also controversial. In her comprehensive review of the literature on flexibility, Harris[3] claimed that in many cases a single measure of flexibility has been used to assess an individual's flexibility characteristics. She concluded, however, that there was no evidence that a single measure can represent a general characteristic of the human body. Others agree that a test such as the sit-and-reach test, which measures trunk and hip flexion (see Chapter 7), is a fairly accurate indicator of an individual's flexibility, since it involves movement in the many joints of the spine and in the hip joints as well.

Properties of Connective Tissue That Affect Joint Flexibility

The range of movement at a joint is determined by the extensibility of the muscles, the elasticity of the articular capsules, the fluidity of the disks, the extensibility of the joint bones (articulations), and the resistance of the surrounding tissues. Kottke, Pauley, and Petak[4] reported that clinical observation has shown that collagenous tissue, which is common in ligaments and tendons, has the property of shortening in the absence of tension as well as the property of plasticity—it slowly elongates under moderate constant tension. They claimed that connective tissue has a very high tensile resistance to suddenly applied tension of short duration. Under prolonged mild tension, however, it elongates. Kottke et al. attributed this elongation to the separation of adjacent collagen fibers. They claimed that normal motion in joints and soft tissue—joint capsules, muscles, subcutaneous tissue, and ligaments—is maintained by the normal movement of the parts of the body, which elongate and stretch these tissues many times each day.

It has been claimed that the major components of joint stiffness are elasticity and plasticity. Researchers have found pronounced age and sex differences in elastic stiffness[5]. Subjects in the sixth decade of life were ten times stiffer than those in the first decade, and a significant increase in elastic stiffness was found in males. Girls have been found to be more flexible than boys, but this difference tends to disappear after puberty. Figure 3.2 shows differences in trunk flexibility, by age and sex, based on a recent fitness survey of more than 15,000 individuals.

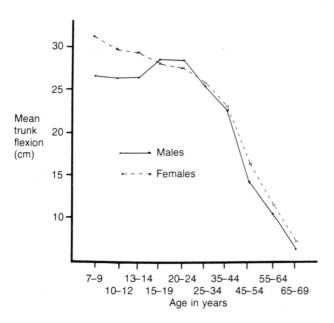

FIGURE 3.2 Trunk flexibility, by age and sex. *Source: Canada's Fitness*, June 1982 survey of Fitness and Amateur Sport, Ottawa. Used by permission.

Responses of Intact Muscle to Stretch

Muscle-stretching techniques are limited by several physiological factors, among them the autogenetic stretch reflex[6]. This mechanism, also known as the myotatic reflex, has been studied for almost 100 years. When stretch is applied to a muscle it causes the muscle fibers to lengthen, which normally excites the annulospiral receptor organs (muscle spindles) within the muscle. This excitation results in monosynaptic stimulation of the efferent motoneurons, which in turn causes the muscle to contract. At the same time that the stretch reflex transmits impulses that excite the stretched muscle, inhibitory impulses are transmitted to the motoneurons of the antagonist muscles. This suggests that local muscle stretch may result in widespread complex changes about the joint involved. A *tonic* stretch reflex is caused by a continuous stretch and is normally weak; a *phasic* stretch reflex is caused by a sudden increase in stretch and is a strong reflex.

It has been well established that in humans a relaxed muscle is electrically silent. The evidence is less conclusive, however, on the question of whether there is a neuromuscular response when passive (tonic) or active (phasic) stretch is applied to muscle. The premise that human intact muscle, when stretched passively, elicits a stretch reflex similar to the response obtained by researchers using excised and treated muscles from laboratory animals, has led to much investigation since the advent of electromyography. Studies in which electromyography was used to examine reflex muscle activity during passive movement (mechanical or manual stretching or shortening) of an intact muscle have shown that little or no activity was present in the muscle.

Effects of Exercise on Joint Flexibility

Exercise programs in physical education, athletics, aerospace medicine, and therapeutics have been directed towards improved human efficiency and performance. Impairment of mobility due to shortening or fixation of connective tissue can result in decreases in muscular strength and endurance. Kottke, Pauley, and Petak claimed that sitting and standing may produce fatigue rapidly if a normally balanced posture cannot be assumed due to impairment of mobility. Fatigued muscles can exert less tension, which is the main stimulus for maintaining strength. The consequent loss of mobility initiates a cycle of muscular deconditioning: reduced muscular activity leads to further impairment of motion, which in turn leads to still further deconditioning[7]. This cycle can be reversed through exercise.

Exercises for the development or maintenance of flexibility are of two types: passive and active. Passive exercise can be divided into nonforced and forced movement. Nonforced movement takes place within the existing voluntary range of motion. It does not cause pain or spasm and has been found to assist in the prevention of contractures, adhesions, capsular tightness, and muscle shortening. Forced passive exercise is carried beyond the voluntary range of motion[8].

Active exercise may be classified as static or kinetic. Static exercise is performed when the muscles contract isometrically without producing joint motion. Kinetic (or dynamic) exercise occurs when muscles contract, producing single or multiple joint movement. This type of exercise may be performed with or without resistance.

Researchers have also investigated the phenomenon of joint flexibility. However, a number of discrepancies and uncertainties still exist in both the literature on and the practice of maintaining and/or increasing the range of joint motion; techniques advocated and practiced vary considerably. Krusen, Kottke, and Ellwood claimed that prolonged moderate stretching is more effective than momentary vigorous stretching[9]. However, a tight muscle can be stretched vigorously as long as it is not inflamed, in which case it ought not be stretched. They also claimed that stretching must be held within one's level of pain tolerance. According to Jensen and Fisher, the best approach to the development of flexibility is to place the tissues on stretch, hold the position for a few seconds, and repeat these two steps several times[10]. They claimed that the slow stretch is both safer and more effective than the bobbing technique, which they do not recommend. Some researchers claim that a quick movement does not stretch out a muscle, whereas a strong, sustained pull does. Others argue that a series of small bouncing motions in which the muscle is forced into more and more stretch improves flexibility.

Flexibility can be increased effectively by means of static stretching and/or slow intermittent stretching. Reid compared these techniques, applying an equal force with each one[11]. Although the intermittent force developed a greater range of joint motion in the first few minutes than the static force, after 10 minutes there was no difference in the amount of flexibility developed.

THE MUSCULAR SYSTEM

Structure of Muscle

The source of power for body movement comes from highly specialized cells or fibers grouped into organs called muscles. Each fiber can perform work by transforming chemical energy into mechanical energy. This process is controlled by the nervous system. Let us examine in simple terms the structure and function of the muscular system.

Skeletal muscle is usually attached to the periosteum of a bone, at its origin and insertion, by muscle tendons (Figure 3.3). It normally traverses one or more joints of the body, so that when it is active it can stabilize or produce movement at the joints.

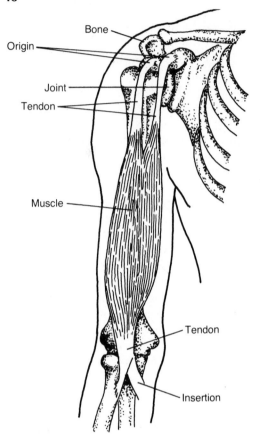

FIGURE 3.3
A typical muscle, showing gross
anatomical structures.

Removal of the skin, fat, and superficial fascia around a muscle would
expose its outer cover or sheath of connective tissue—the *epimysium*. This sheath
blends at each end of the muscle with its tendons. Within the epimysium are
bundles of fibers, or *fasciculi,*consisting of anywhere from a few to thousands
of fibers. Each fasciculus has its own sheath, or *perimysium.* Figure 3.4 illustrates
these structures, which are large enough to be seen without magnification.

Each muscle fiber has an outer connective sheath called the *endomysium.*
Since many muscle fibers do not run the full length of the muscle, these connective
sheaths attach to the other connective sheaths of the muscle—the perimysium
and the epimysium—so that tension may be transmitted the full length of the
muscle.

The muscle cell or fiber is multinucleate, has a diameter up to that of a
human hair, and varies in length from a few centimeters to over 30 centimeters.
Each fiber can be stimulated by a nervous impulse, depolarizing the cell membrane and resulting in the fiber contracting.

Within the *sarcolemma,* the thin membrane that surrounds the muscle
fiber, are many nuclei, mitochrondria, and other intracellular proteins suspended
in sarcoplasm. Within each muscle cell, running longitudinally in rows, are thin

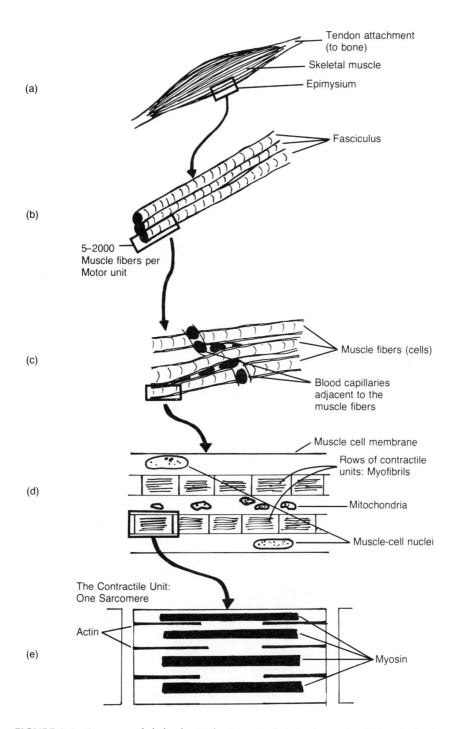

(a)

Tendon attachment
(to bone)

Skeletal muscle

Epimysium

(b)

Fasciculus

5–2000
Muscle fibers per
Motor unit

(c)

Muscle fibers (cells)

Blood capillaries
adjacent to the
muscle fibers

(d)

Muscle cell membrane

Rows of contractile
units: Myofibrils

Mitochondria

Muscle-cell nuclei

(e)

The Contractile Unit:
One Sarcomere

Actin

Myosin

FIGURE 3.4 Structure of skeletal muscle: (a) typical skeletal muscle; (b) longitudinal rows composed of motor units that make up a skeletal muscle; (c) rows of muscle fibers within a motor unit; (d) interior of a muscle cell, with rows of sarcomeres; (e) a sarcomere (the contractile unit), with myosin and actin proteins.

19

myofibrils, which actually contract the muscle. Each myofibril is composed of many contractile units called *sarcomeres;* within each sarcomere are contractile proteins, *myosin* and *actin.* It is within the myofibrils that the energy within food is converted into mechanical energy, which in turn produces work (see Chapter 5).

The Motor Unit

The functional unit of skeletal muscle is the motor unit. It consists of a number of fibers, each supplied with a nerve branch from one motor neuron. There are thousands of motor units in each muscle, and from a few to a few thousand muscle fibers in each motor unit. Muscles that produce precise, delicate movements such as those controlling movement of the eyeballs have very few fibers per motor unit. In contrast, the powerful muscles, such as the gastrocnemius, that thrust the body upward in jumping or forward and upward in running, have been found to contain as many as 2000 fibers per motor unit. A stimulus arrives at a motor unit through its motor neuron. If it is strong enough, all the muscle fibers within that motor unit contract simultaneously. A vigorous contraction of a muscle such as the gastrocnemius appears smooth even though it involves the contraction of a considerable number of motor units. This is because the motor units are stimulated asynchronously and contract up to 50 times per second. Furthermore, the muscle fibers of a motor unit are spread out within the muscle and intermingle with the fibers of other motor units.

Types of Muscular Contraction

Contraction of muscle occurs when action potentials traveling along motor neurons are strong enough to elicit a response from muscle fibers within motor units. This development of tension within the muscle results in a tendency for the muscle to shorten. Although muscles may shorten, lengthen, or remain the same length when active, they always pull on their attachments (origins and insertions); muscles cannot push. There are two types of muscular contractions: isometric and isotonic (Figure 3.5).

Isometric Contraction.   This type of contraction, also called static contraction, occurs when tension develops within a muscle and no noticeable movement occurs at the joints associated with the muscle. In other words, the muscle develops tension but its length remains constant.

Isotonic Contraction.   This type of contraction is often called dynamic contraction. It occurs when tension develops within a muscle and there is a corresponding shortening or lengthening of the muscle. When an active muscle shortens, the isotonic contraction is called concentric contraction. An example of this is shown in Figure 3.5: the elbow flexors contract and shorten, flexing the elbow joint and thereby lifting the mass held in the hand. If the load is

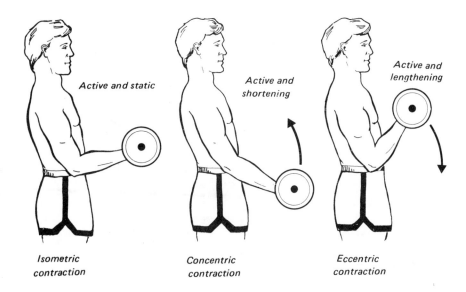

Active and static

Active and
shortening

Active and
lengthening

Isometric
contraction

Concentric
contraction

Eccentric
contraction

FIGURE 3.5 Types of contractions of active muscle. *Source*: James G. Hay and
J. Gavin Reid, *The Anatomical and Mechanical Bases of Human Motion* © 1982,
p. 43. Reprinted by permission of Prentice-Hall, Inc., Englewood Cliffs, N.J.

lowered slowly (under control), the same muscle group is active, but now the
muscles, although still developing tension, are lengthening. This form of isotonic
contraction is called eccentric contraction. It is a common type of contraction,
occurring, for example, when one lowers a mass (Figure 3.5) or walks down
stairs.

Muscular Strength and Endurance

It is important to differentiate between muscular strength and muscular
endurance. *Muscular strength* is the amount of tension that a muscle or muscle
group can exert in a single maximum contraction. Normally it is measured as
an isometric contraction, in which the muscle can generate its maximum tension.
However, it can now be accurately measured isotonically (both concentric and
eccentric contractions) by sophisticated equipment. *Muscular endurance*, on the
other hand, is the capacity of a muscle or muscle group to sustain a contraction
for a certain period of time or to perform continuous work.

A test for muscular strength involves the measurement of a single maximum
contraction. A test for muscular endurance, on the other hand, requires the
measurement of repeated contractions.

Effects of Exercise on Muscle

Muscular Hypertrophy. One of the most obvious effects of a strength-exercise
program on an individual is the increase in the size of the muscles exercised.

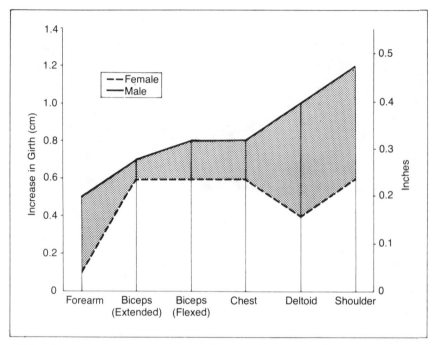

FIGURE 3.6 Increase in muscle size (hypertrophy) is generally not as great in females as in males, even when the same relative gains in strength have been made. *Source*: Edward L. Fox, *Lifetime Fitness.* Copyright © 1983 by CBS College Publishing. Reprinted by permission of Holt, Rinehart and Winston, CBS College Publishing.

More specifically, this hypertrophy of muscle is an enlargement of the cross-sectional area of the muscle and its connective tissues; it results from an enlargement of the myofibrils and of the capillaries supplying each muscle fiber. Increased muscle bulk is often regarded as desirable by men but is thought to be less desirable by women. It has been reported, however, that when men and women perform strength exercises that result in similar gains in strength, the women's muscles do not generally hypertrophy as much as the men's (Figure 3.6). The difference may be a result of fat-tissue loss, initial strength, or changes in muscle bulk.

Hypertrophy of muscle due to increased strength through exercises can be compatible with flexibility. It is a myth that muscle hypertrophy resulting from weight training causes muscle-boundness and immobility. This occurs only over a long period of time and only if the training does not allow the full range of joint motion or does not include flexibility exercises.

The Overload Principle. To develop strength effectively, one should follow the overload principle: in exercising, use work loads or resistances that are greater than those normally used. The greater the percentage of a muscle's maximum strength that is utilized during training, the greater will be the strength development over time. One is best able to gain strength, therefore, through heavy-resistance exercises that incorporate the use of weights.

The Principle of Progressive Resistance. Muscle that is exercised according to the overload principle will increase its strength within a few weeks. The load that was used during this period is handled more easily now and is therefore insufficient to effectively develop further strength. At this stage the resistance should be increased, on the basis of the overload principle. The exercise then resumes and further gains in strength are thus made possible.

The Principle of Specificity. Specificity of training is a well-accepted principle. There are little or no benefits to be gained in muscular endurance, for instance from a program designed to improve muscular strength. If weight-training exercises for the development of strength in a muscle or muscle group are performed correctly, the resulting increase in strength may be considerable while the improvement in muscular endurance may be negligible. On the other hand, endurance training of leg muscles for, say, long-distance running will have a minimal effect on the strength of those muscles.

Antigravity Musculature

The maintenance of an erect stance during locomotion depends upon control of the musculoskeletal system not only by the conscious activity of the brain but also by righting reflexes. Some of these righting reflexes are neuromuscular: they consist of nervous impulses initiated by stretch receptors (proprioceptive mechanisms) within the skeletal muscles. Others, such as the optical righting reflexes, depend on vision. Still others—labyrinthine righting reflexes—depend on mechanisms that detect position and change.

The muscle groups that are responsible for maintaining erect posture—and, more generally, for holding the joints of the body in extension—are called antigravity muscles. These muscle groups are shown in Figure 3.7. Not all of them are active when a person maintains an erect stance, but they would become active if the individual's balance were disrupted.

Muscle Groups

The exercise specialist should be qualified to prescribe exercises and activities for the development of strength and endurance in all the major muscles of the body. Since there are approximately 500 muscles in the body, this would be a mammoth task unless the major muscles were sorted into groups. For simplicity's sake, the muscles are grouped according to their actions on the joints of the body. For example, the muscles responsible for active flexion of the cervical vertebrae (the sternocleidomastoids) are called the neck flexors: the three muscles

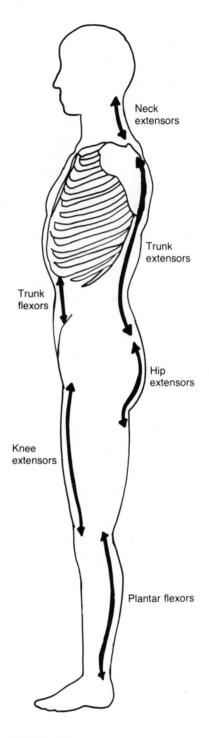

FIGURE 3.7
Antigravity muscles. (The trunk flexors are often not included in this group.)

TABLE 3.1   Major Joints and Associated Movements for Exercise Prescription

JOINTS	MOVEMENTS
Neck	flexion, extension, rotation, lateral bending
Trunk	flexion, extension, rotation, lateral bending
Shoulder girdle	abduction, adduction, elevation, depression
Shoulder joint	flexion, extension, abduction, adduction, rotation, horizontal abduction and adduction
Elbow	flexion, extension
Wrist	flexion, extension
Hip	flexion, extension, abduction, adduction, rotation, horizontal abduction and adduction
Knee	flexion, extension
Ankle	plantar flexion, dorsiflexion

that flex the shoulder joint (the pectoralis major, deltoid, and coracobrachialis) are the shoulder flexors; and the muscles that cause plantar flexion of the ankle joint (gastrocnemius, soleus, and plantaris) are called the plantar flexors. The major joints of the body and the possible actions or movements at those joints are presented in Table 3.1.

REFERENCES

1. James G. Hay and J. Gavin Reid, *The Anatomical and Mechanical Bases of Human Motion* (Englewood Cliffs, N.J.: Prentice-Hall, 1982), p. 33.
2. Robert L. Larson, "Physical Activity and the Growth and Development of Bone and Joint Structures," in *Physical Activity Human Growth and Development,* ed. G. L. Rarick (New York: Academic Press, 1973), pp. 32–59.
3. Margaret L. Harris, "Flexibility: Review of the Literature," *American Physical Therapy,* 49 (June 1969), 591–601.
4. Frederic J. Kottke, Donna L. Pauley, and Rudolph A. Petak, "The Rationale for Prolonged Stretching and Correction of Shortening of Connective Tissue," *Archives of Physical Medicine and Rehabilitation,* 47 (June 1966), 347.
5. Verna Wright and Richard J. Johns, "Observations on the Measurement of Joint Stiffness," *Arthritis and Rheumatism,* 3 (August 1960), 328.
6. George J. Holland, "The Physiology of Flexibility: A Review of the Literature," in *Kinesiology Review* (Washington, D.C.: American Association for Health, Physical Education and Recreation, 1968), pp. 49–62.
7. Kottke, Pauley, and Petak, "Rationale for Prolonged Stretching," pp. 345–52.
8. Janet A. Wessel and Wayne Van Huss, "Therapeutic Aspects of Exercise in Medicine," in *Science and Medicine of Exercise and Sports,* ed. Warren R. Johnson (New York: Harper, 1960), p. 672.
9. F. H. Krusen, F. J. Kottke, and P. M. Ellwood, *Handbook for Physical Medicine and Rehabilitation* (Philadelphia: Saunders, 1971).
10. Clayne R. Jensen and A. Garth Fisher, *Scientific Basis of Athletic Conditioning,* 2nd ed. (Philadelphia: Lea & Febiger, 1979), p. 205.
11. J. Gavin Reid, "Effects of Constant and Intermittent Forces on Range of Joint Motion," in *Biomechanics V-A,* ed. P. V. Komi, International Series on Biomechanics, vol. 1A (Baltimore: University Park Press, 1976), pp. 461–67.

4

Human Posture: Structure and Dynamics

INTRODUCTION

Human posture, or body mechanics, although of general concern to the vast majority of people, has been a subject of practical and scientific interest to anatomists, anthropologists, orthopedic surgeons, psychiatrists, physical educators, (kinesiologists), and many other specialists. The tissues of the body have been studied in detail by the anatomist; the evolution of the body and variations in it due to race and habitat have been researched by the anthropologist; structural defects in the body have been a focus of the orthopedic surgeon; the relationship of posture to mental and social stresses has been studied by the psychiatrist; and efficient human motion and the prescription of exercise to restore, maintain, and/or improve fitness have been concerns of the physical educator. Although these specialists have different skills and interests, their knowledge of human posture overlaps. A common area of interest is the development of the spine.

The spine of the human fetus and newborn has a single primary curve in the sagittal plane (Figure 4.1a). The initial secondary curve appears in the cervical region (neck) of the very pliable spinal column of the one-to-two-months-old child (Figure 4.1b). This curve is due to the development of the neck extensors, which the prone child uses to raise its head so that it can look around. The next secondary curve appears in the lumbar region (Figure 4.1c). It is due to devel-

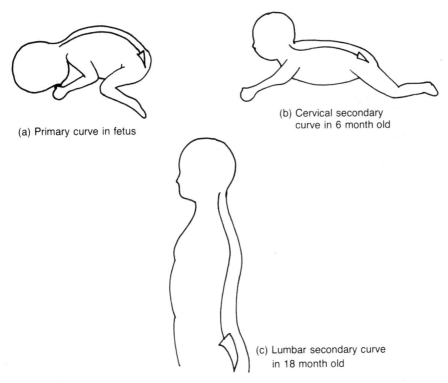

(a) Primary curve in fetus

(b) Cervical secondary curve in 6 month old

(c) Lumbar secondary curve in 18 month old

FIGURE 4.1 Primary and secondary curves of the spinal column.

opment of the trunk-extensor muscles, which results from the antigravity muscular activity performed during crawling and sitting up and from the resistance of the hip flexors across the hip joints. There are two other primary spinal curves—the thoracic and the sacrococcygeal curves. The resistance of the hip flexors, in particular the psoas and the iliacus, to total hip and lumbar-vertebrae extension is illustrated in Figure 4.2. The development of the hip extensors, which provide erect posture when they are extended at the hip joints, causes a simultaneous forward traction in the lumbar region that is commonly referred to as lumbar lordosis[1]. During their first few years of growth children usually show a rather pronounced lumbar lordosis, which sometimes remains throughout life but more commonly decreases considerably.

This knowledge is vitally important to anyone concerned with the prescription of exercise, because physical activity has not only a modifying effect on the structure of the body but often social and psychological consequences as well. The importance of understanding the structure and dynamics of human posture cannot be overemphasized. The exercise prescriptionist must be able to carefully *observe* the relationship of an individual's body parts; *assess* whether that individual's body mechanics are sound or whether there is a malalignment of body parts; *decide* whether specific exercises need to be prescribed; *select*

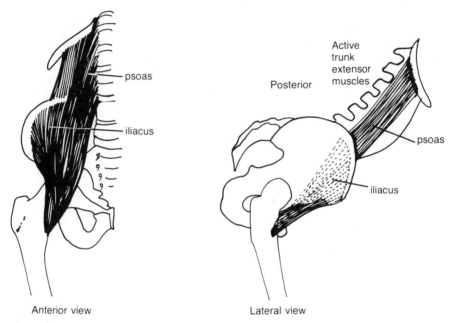

Anterior view   Lateral view

FIGURE 4.2   Resistance of iliacus and iliopsoas to trunk extension results in lumbar curve development.

suitable exercises for the individual; *teach* the individual how to perform the exercises; and, finally, *evaluate* the effects of the prescribed exercises.

Posture has been defined as the "relative arrangement of the different parts . . . of the body: . . . the position or bearing of the body [as a whole] whether characteristic or assumed for a special purpose"[2]. Any definition of human posture should consider the proper alignment or relationship of the various body segments.

In recumbency and erect standing, the body is in a state of rest and almost no movement occurs, although there is constant adjustment of body parts. These two positions are sometimes referred to as static posture. Dynamic posture, on the other hand, consists of movements such as walking, running, climbing stairs, and lifting.

ERECT STANDING POSTURE

Steindler[3] suggested that good posture depends essentially on the correctness of two relations: first, the relation between the line of weight and the spinal column; second, the anteroposterior tilt of the pelvis. Figure 4.3 shows the relation of the line of weight to the anteroposterior spinal curves. Note that the line of weight intersects both the cervicothoracic and lumbothoracic junctions.

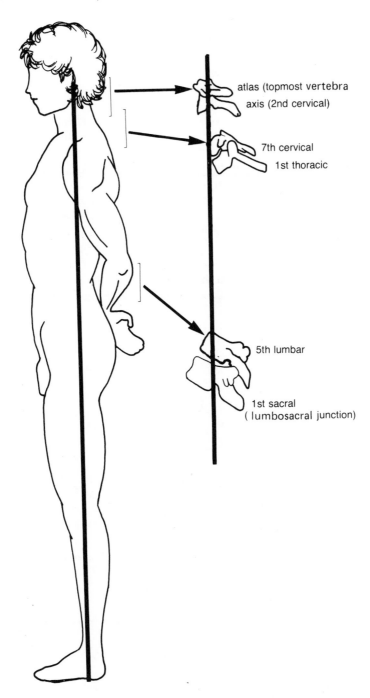

atlas (topmost vertebra
axis (2nd cervical)

7th cervical
1st thoracic

5th lumbar

1st sacral
(lumbosacral junction)

FIGURE 4.3 The line of weight passes through the center of
mass of the body and intersects the joints indicated.

Another element of good posture is the physiologic lumbosacral angle for the static spine (Figure 4.4), which is normally about 30 degrees[4].These and other posture-evaluation methods presented in the literature may well be valuable in the clinical diagnosis of posture malalignment or deviation. However, in the assessment of posture by the exercise specialist they are of limited use because they usually require radiography for observation.

Erect standing posture has been evaluated through the use of many different methods, but it is best defined in terms of the relationship of the parts of the body to the line of weight—a vertical line that passes through the center of mass of the body. The location of the center of mass of the body in the erect standing position will vary somewhat from individual to individual depending on limb length, body-mass distribution, body shape, and posture. In general, however, it has been reported to lie at about 55 to 57 percent of the height of the individual and near the junction of the fifth lumbar and first sacral vertebrae (see Figure 4.3).

The line of weight has a very important relationship to the joints of the body and their axes of rotation. If it lies in front of the joint, there is a tendency for movement to occur at that joint. That tendency, however, may be balanced by counterforces.

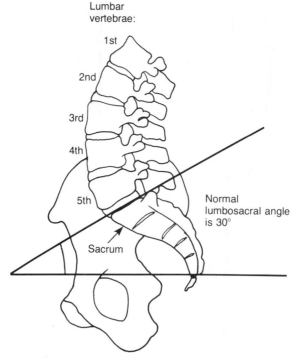

FIGURE 4.4 Physiologic lumbosacral angle.

In the normal erect standing position the line of weight should pass through the head slightly anterior to the atlanto-occipital joints. If we observe a subject along the frontal plane (from the side), as in Figure 4.3, we can see that the line passes through the tragus (lobe) of the ear. Because the line of weight is anterior to the axes of rotation, there is a tendency for the neck to flex and the head to fall forward in the sagittal plane. This action is countered by the neck extensors (see Table A.1 in the Appendix). If the head is habitually held forward—that is, if the line of weight is well forward of the atlanto-occipital joints—undue strain is placed on both the extensor ligaments and muscles in the posterior aspect of the neck. In many societies people customarily carry loads on their heads, which must be perfectly balanced to minimize torque and thus strain. This balancing appears to result in good posture in the upper torso, head, and neck.

Below the atlanto-occipital joints the line of weight intersects the spinal column at the cervicothoracic junction (Figure 4.3), the thoracolumbar articulation, and the lumbosacral joint. It then passes close to the anterior of the sacroiliac joint[5]. If we were to drop a plumb line from the tragus of a person standing in a good erect position, it should pass one to two centimeters posterior to the greater trochanter of the femur. This does not necessarily mean, however, that the subject's posture is good in the spinal region. One has to assess the amount of curve in the spinal column from both a lateral and a posterior viewpoint. The degree of anteroposterior curve will be discussed later in this chapter in the section on the diagnosis of common postural problems.

Figure 4.5 shows the relation of the line of weight to the hip joint in two different situations. In Figure 4.5a the line of weight is anterior to the hip joint. This results in a tendency for the hip joint to become flexed. Flexion in the sagittal plane around a transverse axis will occur unless a counterforce is generated by the contraction of a hip-extensor muscle such as the gluteus maximus. In Figure 4.5b the line of weight is posterior to the hip joint. The result is a tendency for hyperextension of the hip joint. In the erect standing position the hip is usually hyperextended approximately 10 degrees. It would be expected that the counterforce to further hyperextension would be achieved by the contraction of the main hip flexors (the iliopsoas, rectus femoris, pectineus, sartorius, and tensor fasciae latae). Although this premise has been accepted by many writers and researchers, electromyographic studies have found that except for the iliopsoas, which remains quite active in the erect posture[6], the hip flexors are relaxed. The slight hyperextension at the hip joint is maintained predominantly by the iliofemoral ligament, which is located on the medial anterior aspect of the joint. Regarded as the strongest ligament in the body, it becomes taut when the hip is slightly hyperextended and by supporting the hip joint it enables one to stand upright.

From near the greater trochanter of the femur, the line of weight passes close to the patella bones and slightly anterior to the center of rotation (the transverse axes) of the knee joints. When a standing person extends his or her

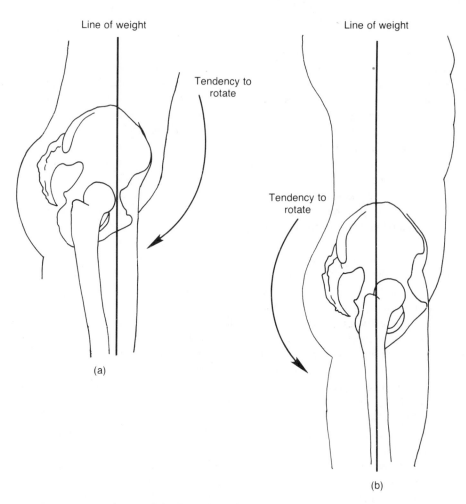

FIGURE 4.5 Relation of the line of weight and the hip joints: (a) line of weight anterior to the axis of rotation tends to cause flexion at the hip joints; (b) line of weight posterior to axis of rotation tends to cause hyperextension at the hip joints.

knee, the femur rotates medially on the tibia. The lateral condyle is almost stationary during this movement, whereas the medial condyle slides backwards. Extension of the knee is completed by a movement that places the knee in a slightly hyperextended position of approximately 5 to 10 degrees. Commonly termed the *screw-home movement* of the knee, this rotary phenomenon is in fact the normal locking action of the knee joint. This locked position allows the quadriceps (the knee-extensor muscles) to relax while the load of the body at the knee joints is being supported by the bony structure and ligaments of the knee. The relaxed state of the quadriceps during erect standing can be shown by use of electromyography. However, the children's trick of unexpectedly pushing a friend's knees from behind is a simple illustration of this phenomenon. This action, together with the relaxed state of the knee extensors, causes a sudden loss of stability. The sudden decent of the body results in the lengthening (stretch) of these extensors, which in turn causes the stretch receptors within the muscles to be stimulated. This stretch reflex results in rapid contraction of the quadriceps, which prevents the person from collapsing.

The line of weight in the erect standing position is distributed fairly equally by the ankle joints to the base of support (the feet). The lines of force pass anterior to the axes of rotation and about midway between the supporting structure of the calcanei (heels) and the heads of the metatarsals, or about 2 to 5 centimeters anterior to the lateral malleoli. Because the line of weight is anterior to the transverse axes of the ankle joints, a torque (rotatory force) is present that will rotate the body forward over the ankles if a counterforce provided by the triceps surae is absent. The most active of this group of muscles (the plantar flexors) during erect standing is the soleus. It can perform the sustained tonic activity required during prolonged standing.

If the line of weight falls outside the base of support, stability is lost and the person will fall or be forced to regain his or her balance. When balance is deliberately disturbed, motion occurs. If controlled, as in walking, stair climbing, and lifting, this motion can be observed and assessed and is regarded as dynamic posture.

DYNAMIC POSTURE

Assessment and improvement of posture are usually directed toward erect standing posture. Equally important in exercise prescription for fitness, but more difficult to assess or quantify, is the dynamic posture involved in sitting, lifting, walking, running and other such physical activities.

Sitting

Sitting for relaxation in a comfortable chair seldom presents problems of posture, since the body parts may be moved as soon as discomfort is experienced. This is often not the case when one is seated in an upright chair or at a bench in a factory and performing work such as typing, writing, or a manual job. Here the individual is confined to a limited area and movement is often restricted for long periods. It is important, therefore, that the trunk and head be held in a comfortable upright position. Slight modifications of the upright seated position should be made fairly frequently.

Good sitting posture depends not only on the individual but upon a well-designed chair and a table or counter top placed at the correct height for him or her. The height and inclination of the chair seat should allow the person to sit comfortably with the hips well back and slightly below the level of the knees. The thighs should therefore be elevated a little at the distal ends and the feet should be placed comfortably on the floor. The edge of the seat should not exert pressure against the back of the knees. The buttocks and thighs should be supported evenly by as large an area as possible so that undue pressure at any one part can be avoided. The back of the chair should support the area of the lumbar vertebrae and permit the individual to sit upright. The table or counter surface should be a little above elbow height so that when the shoulders are slightly flexed the elbows can rest on the surface without elevation or depression of the shoulder girdle.

Lifting

The lifting of objects occurs at home, in the factory, on the streets, and in play, and is also an important part of the exercise scene. It is agreed that the most common hazard to the back is the act of improperly lifting an object from near the floor[7]. This action can create excessive moments about the lumbosacral region that result in increased stress and frequent injury. An understanding of those basic principles of body mechanics that apply to lifting is important not only in performing the activities of daily life but in prescribing exercises involving the movement of heavy masses, such as strength exercises.

When lifting a heavy object from the ground, one should squat so that the object is as close to the center of the body as possible. This will increase one's mechanical advantage in lifting the load. The feet should be comfortably placed flat on the floor close to the mass, and the knees should be bent. The lift should be made with a slow, simultaneous extension of the knees and hips; the back is held relatively straight (Figure 4.6b). Lifting should be performed by the powerful muscles of the legs—the knee and hip extensors—and not by the arms and back.

To reduce the chance of injury to the knees and back while holding a heavy mass, one should slightly flex the knees and avoid hyperextension. The mass should be evenly distributed between both feet when at all possible. One should avoid turning the body while holding the mass, as this action causes increased stress on the joints. Light objects may be lifted by flexion (bending) at the hips. However, those who have a history of lower-back pain should use a correct lifting technique at all times to protect unnecessary strain to the lower back.

Contraction of the abdominal musculature is an important safety factor in the lifting of masses, as during strength exercises. Not only does this action tend to reduce the curve in the lower back (lumbar lordosis) but it makes the trunk into a more solid column, thereby reducing considerably the stresses on the vulnerable intervertebral disks.

Walking

Walking posture is as variable among individuals as is erect standing posture. Differences are due to a large number of factors, many of which are

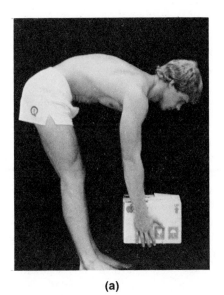 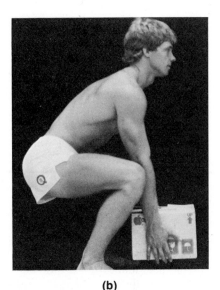

(a)   **(b)**

FIGURE 4.6 Lifting a load: (a) incorrect technique; (b) correct technique—knees and hips flexed, trunk straight and as nearly erect as possible.

similar to those affecting standing posture. They include age and sex, body size, length of body segments and their alignment, distribution of body mass, range of motion at the joints, shape and size of the bones and joints, muscle strength and balance, and the physical and mental health of the individual. Despite these variables, and even though the mechanical and physiological demands of different types of walking—such as strolling, striding, marching, and race walking—also cause noticeable variations in posture, there are certain postural requirements for efficient gait.

Numerous research articles and papers concerned with quantitative and qualitative analysis of human locomotion are available in the literature[8,9,10]. Many of these papers detail factors that affect normal and pathological gait, such as the inclination of the body, the action of the supporting leg, the swinging phase, vertical and rotatory movements of the pelvis, and the contributions of the shoulders, arms, and head. Students interested in the study of walking posture should become familiar with some of these publications.

A simple and brief description of walking is presented here as a way of emphasizing some of the important principles of posture. The trunk and head should be held almost erect, with a slight inclination forward, but as relaxed as possible. The arms should hang freely with minimal rigidity in the shoulder girdle and should swing rhythmically at the sides in the sagittal plane. The legs swing forward alternately. When the heel strikes the ground, the weight of the body moves forward over the lateral side of the foot and then medially to the first toe to complete the supporting phase of that foot. This phase coincides with the swinging phase of the other leg, the heel of which strikes the ground prior to the toe-off action of the supporting leg. There is a short period in which both feet are in contact with the ground. This distinguishes walking from running, in which only one foot is in contact with the ground at a time. The foot should be placed on the ground so that it is facing forward, but moderate deviation (toe in or toe out, the latter being more common) is acceptable.

Running

Running differs from walking in many ways, the most noticeable being the absence of double support (the feet are never in contact with the ground at the same time) and the intervals of nonsupport (periodically both feet are off the ground and the runner is airborne). Running is similar to walking in that it is a form of human locomotion in which the legs and arms both swing alternately. The legs have a support phase and a swing phase, and the arms swing forward and backward from the shoulder joint to maintain balance.

As in walking, the form used in running depends to a large degree upon the physical makeup of the runner. The age, sex, size, length of body segments and their alignment, distribution of mass, flexibility of joints, bone architecture, muscle strength and balance, and physical and mental health all influence running form. Although certain basic mechanical principles can be applied to the running form of all individuals, no two persons will run in an identical manner.

It does not require an experienced eye to observe the very poor running form of many joggers and runners as they pound the sidewalks in and around our cities and towns. Most have been advised, frequently by health professionals, that to improve their cardiovascular and respiratory fitness they should jog or run several kilometers at least three times a week! Seldom do these people receive instruction on running technique, training methods, training surfaces, flexibility, or appropriate clothing and footwear. Running just 5 kilometers 3 times a week will result in the body experiencing approximately 15,000 impacts of the foot on the ground. Incorrect running posture and mechanics can and usually do have a hazardous effect upon one's health. A study of 900 endurance runners revealed that some 18 percent had knee problems, 14 percent achilles tendonitis, 11.6 percent tibial stress syndromes (including stress fracture), 6.9 percent arch injuries, and 4.9 percent foot fractures, all requiring cessation of training for a period [11]. This represents approximately 500 of the 900 runners, an alarming statistic. Exercise prescriptionists should be very careful to inform others on a number of important points when prescribing running or walking for fitness:

1. body mechanics and posture: individual differences in running and walking form
2. training programs: physiological adaptation and individual differences
3. strength and flexibility programs
4. training surfaces and terrain: grass fields such as a golf course are preferable to hard, cambered road and sidewalk surfaces
5. quality footwear: selected for maximum protection and shock absorbency
6. weather conditions: excessive heat and cold should both be avoided

As in walking, there are certain basic mechanical principles of form that should be considered by all people who run. During steady running, the body should be relaxed but held erect, the chest out and the abdomen held in comfortably. There should be a slight forward lean, especially when one is running against the wind. The head should be aligned with the trunk and facing forward. As much as possible, running should be done in a straight line, the feet making contact with the ground below or slightly in front of the runner and the toes pointed forward. To reduce the impact of the foot on the ground, one should make contact with the outer border of the ball of the foot and follow this with a slight pronation (inversion) of the foot as the heel makes contact. Two forms of running that should be avoided are making contact first with the heel and running only on the ball of the foot.

CAUSES OF POOR POSTURE

Postural defects have many different causes; often a single defect is attributed to one or more causes. Causes may be classified as medical or psychiatric on the one hand or nonpathological on the other, and a defect may well be associated with causes in both groups.

Medical or Psychiatric Causes

These include diseases that prevent natural growth of bones and joints and weaken both the skeletal and muscular systems. Loss of strength in specific muscles results in muscular imbalance and malalignment of body parts. Attitude and emotions also influence posture and movement. Erect posture is often related to feelings of elation and confidence; slumping posture is very much associated with depression or feelings of inadequacy. It is most important in dealing with children in the latter state to rebuild their self-esteem before the poor posture becomes habitual.

Injury to bones, joints, and muscles usually weakens the affected area, and if the injury is to a supportive structure, it may well cause malalignment and imbalance. Prolonged casting of a limb as a result of a break to a bone such as the tibia often leaves the person with an unnatural gait. The person is usually not aware of the habit, and thus the relearning of movement skills is most important in his or her rehabilitation.

Nonpathological Causes

These causes of poor posture are many and variable. They include improper clothing (too tight or heavy); shoes that are poorly designed and constructed, such as high heels; physical defects (for example, legs of different length); defective hearing and/or vision; poor nutrition (underweight or obesity); furniture design not related to user's size or needs; heredity; habit; constant use of one side of the body, such as always carrying loads in the same hand; lack of knowledge about posture; and muscular weakness.

The exercise prescriptionist must be aware of these various causes when assessing posture. Removal of the cause does not always correct the ailment, but many postural defects can be corrected by exercise, surgery, or other means.

DIAGNOSIS OF COMMON POSTURAL PROBLEMS

Postural deviations are classified as functional and structural. Functional disorders normally consist of a malalignment of body parts that involves muscle and ligaments; carefully prescribed exercises can correct the disorder. Persisting functional disorders usually become structural, in that the bones adapt to the stresses of malalignment and the deviation becomes permanent. Surgery, bracing, or some other treatment apart from exercise is necessary for the correction of structural defects.

Many postural faults are due to poor muscular development. Children who are physically inactive, and therefore not physiologically fit, are prone to poor posture since muscular strength and endurance are required to maintain good static and dynamic posture for prolonged periods. The "fatigue slump" commonly found in children is due to poor muscular strength and endurance, and results in forward pelvic tilt, pronounced lumbar lordosis, excessive thoracic kyphosis, round shoulders, and forward head. These and other common postural deviations will be discussed below. Knowing how to correct them is very important for anyone prescribing exercises.

It must be emphasized that normality is usually regarded as a standard that represents groups of individuals. There are many variations in posture within any group of individuals, however, and the standard should remain flexible. A slight deviation from the norm might well be suited to an individual; if so, attempts to correct the condition should be avoided unless the exercise prescriptionist is very experienced in dealing with postural deviations. Only when a deviation is functional and noticeable or is extreme enough to affect the efficiency of the systems of the body and/or predispose the individual to discomfort or injury should extra concern be shown.

Forward Head

In this condition the head and neck are held in a forward and slightly downward position with the chin held comfortably in towards the neck (Figure 4.7). This position differs from poke neck, in which the chin is held well away from the neck and an excessive cervical lordosis is present. The former position usually responds well to corrective exercise; the latter, associated very often with nearsightedness, is more difficult to correct.

Line of weight

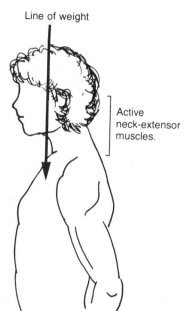

Active
neck-extensor
muscles.

FIGURE 4.7
Forward head: the line of weight is well forward
of the axis of rotation, resulting in much activity
of the neck-extensor muscles to maintain the
position.

The mass of the head is supported mainly by the rather thin cervical vertebrae, and if it is displaced anteriorily, as in forward head, continuous muscular activity of the extensor muscles of the neck is required. This malalignment may result in muscle spasms in the neck, often accompanied by headaches. Apart from that, the position is not aesthetically pleasing.

Round Shoulders

This condition is very often associated with forward head. The shoulders are forward and downward, and the *acromions* (bony processes on the superior/lateral aspect of the scapulae, or shoulder blades) are anterior to the line of weight. The scapulae are abducted, and the medial or vertebral borders and the inferior angles are often pronounced. If the shoulders can be drawn back voluntarily, the condition is considered functional and exercises can be prescribed for strengthening and shortening the shoulder adductors (the rhomboids and lower trapezius muscles). Careful stretching of the scapula depressors (pectoralis minor muscles) will further facilitate the correction. If the shoulders cannot be actively or passively brought back to a normal position, the condition is probably structural and may well be due to abnormally short clavicles. No attempt should be made to correct this condition by prescribing exercises.

Round Back (Kyphosis)

This defect consists of an increased curve in the vertebral column in the thoracic region. In functional kyphosis, the trunk-extensor muscles in the thoracic region can be strengthened as a corrective measure. This is done to best advantage during the preadolescent and adolescent stages of growth.

Lumbar Lordosis

This condition, commonly known as hollow back, is an exaggeration of the normal vertebral curve in the lumbar region (Figure 4.8). Lumbar lordosis is often accompanied by kyphosis and invariably by an increased forward tilt of the pelvic girdle. The condition is often attributed to muscular imbalance. The trunk flexors or fixators (particularly the rectus abdominis) are much weaker anteriorly than the trunk extensors (erector spinae) and the powerful hip flexors (for example, the iliopsoas). The increased slackness in the trunk flexors that insert on the symphysis pubis permit the pelvis to tilt downward. The trunk extensors and the posterior ligaments in the lumbar region become short and tight, thereby maintaining or increasing the height of the superior aspect of the back of the sacrum. In addition, an increased lumbar curve, with the line of weight behind it, lessens the space between the spinal processes and at the same time decreases the size of the vertebral spaces (foramina) through which the spinal nerves pass. After physical activity involving repeated impacts on a hard surface, pressure on these nerves may cause muscular spasms in the lower back or referred pain down the legs.

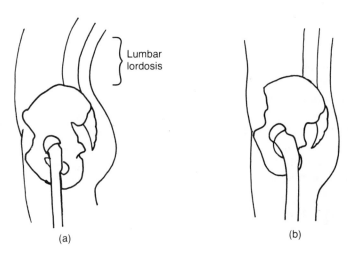

Lumbar
lordosis

(a)   (b)

FIGURE 4.8   Lumbar lordosis: (a) exaggerated curve in the lumbar region; (b) the normal curve.

Flat Back

This is an abnormal decrease in the anteroposterior curves of the spine, in particular the lumbar vertebrae. It is usually accompanied by a decrease in the forward inclination of the pelvis. This rotated position of the pelvis is in the direction opposite to that associated with lumbar lordosis.

Pelvic Tilt

Pelvic tilt in the sagittal plane is either forward or backward. Forward tilting of the pelvis beyond the normal position increases the lumbosacral angle (Figure 4.4). The greater this angle, the greater the shearing stress and the greater the tendency for the fifth lumbar vertebra to slide forward on the sacrum. Forward pelvic tilt is usually exaggerated when a person suffers from visceral ptosis—a prominent abdomen due to an increase in mass resulting from excess fat. Backward tilting of the pelvis, which is associated with flat back, decreases the shock-absorbing qualities of the spinal column and pelvic girdle.

Scoliosis

The word *scoliosis* means twisting or bending, and the condition consists of the lateral bending and longitudinal rotation of the spine in a person standing

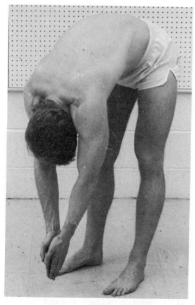

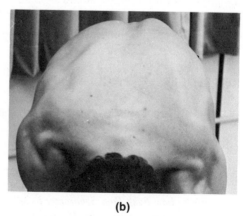

(b)

(a)

FIGURE 4.9 Test for scoliosis: (a) subject in test position; (b) a nonsymmetric back indicating scoliosis.

erect. Prevalent in early adolescence, it begins with a single C curve, convex to the left, and may progress to an S curve if it becomes structural.

Most people have a slight lateral bend to their spine. This is due to muscular imbalance resulting from movement habits such as always using one's dominant side for carrying, throwing, and kicking. Although the exercise specialist should be aware of these habits and attempt to educate people about them, detection of scoliosis in the young and referral of afflicted children to a physician are more important.

There is a simple test for the detection of scoliosis. The subject, shirtless or clad in a light T-shirt, bends forward with hands together and arms straight, as shown in Figure 4.9a. Whereas a normal back is symmetrical, a scoliotic spine will have a noticeable hump on one side of the thoracic and/or lumbar regions (Figure 4.9b). No corrective exercises should be prescribed for an adolescent with scoliosis unless the child's physician refers him or her back to the exercise specialist for treatment.

Leg and Foot

Alignments of the legs and feet are as varied as the gait patterns among individuals. The six most common deviations or defects in the lower limbs are *genu valgum* (knock-knee), *genu varum* (bowlegs), excessively hyperextended knees, tibial torsion, *pes cavus* (high arch in the foot), and *pes planus* (flatfoot). Unless permission or prescription has been given to the exercise specialist by the physician, no attempt should be made to prescribe exercises for these conditions. They often relate one to another, and if they seriously inhibit a person's efficiency, he or she should consult an orthopedic specialist.

REFERENCES

1. Rene Cailliet, *Low Back Pain Syndrome,* 2nd ed. (Philadelphia: F. A. Davis, 1968), p. 14.

2. *Webster's Seventh New Collegiate Dictionary* (Springfield, Mass.: Merriam, 1967), p. 664.

3. Arthur Steindler, *Kinesiology of the Human Body Under Normal and Pathological Conditions* (Springfield, Ill.: Chas. C Thomas, 1955), p. 227.

4. Cailliet, *Low Back Pain Syndrome,* p. 34.

5. Steindler, *Kinesiology of the Human Body,* p. 228.

6. John V. Basmajian, *Muscles Alive: Their Functions Revealed by Electromyography,* 4th ed. (Baltimore: Williams & Wilkins, 1978), p. 182.

7. Don B. Chaffin, "Occupational Biomechanics of Low Back Injury," in *Symposium on Idiopathic Low Back Pain,* ed. A. A. White III and S. L. Gordon (St. Louis: C. V. Mosby, 1982), pp. 323–30.

8. *Human Locomotion I,* Proceedings of the Special Conference of the Canadian Society for Biomechanics, London, Ontario, 1980, pp. 1–137.

9. *Human Locomotion II,* Proceedings of the Second Biannual Conference of the Canadian Society for Biomechanics, Kingston, Ontario, 1982, pp. 1–115.

10. Kit Vaughan, *Biomechanics of Human Gait: An Annotated Bibliography 1873–1981* (Cape Town, South Africa: Department of Biomedical Engineering, University of Cape Town, 1982).

11. Douglas B. Clement and Jack E. Taunton, "Running Induced Injuries to Athletes," *Track and Field Journal,* 1 (February 1980), 6.

5

Muscle Energetics

INTRODUCTION

Exercising the large-muscle groups of the body creates an elevated demand for energy within the working muscle cells. In turn, coordinated and sequential responses to this demand are set into motion throughout almost every system and part of the body. From the brain to the furthest extremities, neural, physiological, and biochemical activity becomes highly elevated. Several of these responses are very important for the improvement of one's fitness, and most are advantageous for the general health and functioning of the body. For these health benefits to accrue, however, large-muscle activity must be performed correctly, with regularity, and at the appropriate intensity.

In Chapter 3 we described the muscle sarcomere, the myosin and actin proteins, and muscular contraction. In this chapter we will discuss the energy demands created by exercise. We hope thereby to help the exercise prescriptionist gain an understanding of the energy demands of various activities and to make intelligent decisions regarding the type, the amount, and the regularity of an exercise regimen. A prerequisite to our discussion is an understanding of the physiology of large-muscle activity, for it is this activity that initiates the demand for energy. In turn, these demands force physiological systems within the body to function at an elevated metabolism—the actual goal of fitness prescription.

When large-muscle activity is performed optimally and with regularity, these physiological systems will experience an improvement in function and capacity. This entire sequence of events is termed *physical fitness*.

THE EXTERNAL SOURCE OF ENERGY FOR THE BODY: FOOD

The source of energy for physical activity as well as for *cellular metabolism* (the healthy maintenance of *all* living tissues in the body) is the foods we consume, principally their carbohydrates and fats. Anyone who daily consumes a balanced diet (discussed at length in Chapter 6) has enough stored energy to perform as much exercise and activity as he or she desires. The energy in food—actually it is locked within the bonding structure of the carbohydrate and fat molecules (see Figure 5.1)—is measured in *calories,* the most commonly understood energy unit for food. Even though this basic unit of energy is quite small, our caloric (food) need is also relatively small, certainly much less so than the majority of North Americans believe.

After a meal has been eaten the carbohydrates and fats are ingested through the gut and eventually either stored or, during exercise, delivered to the working muscle cells. This biochemical processing and transporting of the carbohydrates and fats within the body requires a multitude of physiological activities (also discussed in some detail in Chapter 6). This chapter focuses mainly on the disposition of these carbohydrates and fats once they have reached the working muscles and the production of energy from them. The potential energy contained in the carbohydrate and fat molecules inside muscle cells cannot be utilized directly. First it must be transformed by a sequence of biochemical reactions into the only energy source that the actin and myosin (contractile proteins) in the muscle can utilize: adenosine triphosphate, or ATP (see Figure 5.1). This transformation is carried out by many enzymes—specialized proteins in the muscle cell. The entire enzymatic process is analogous to the refinement of gasoline: although crude oil possesses vast amounts of energy when it is pumped out of the ground, a car's engine cannot utilize this potential energy until it has been refined into a more combustible form.

THE SOURCES OF ATP WITHIN MUSCLE: CAPACITIES AND CHARACTERISTICS

An understanding of the energy sources that are available within the muscle cells is essential in order to first appreciate what types of exercise demand energy from specific source(s), then to understand the resulting physiological reaction of the body, for some activities can prove too stressful, even injurious, while others are too mild. Within the muscle cell there are two main enzyme systems

I. PRODUCTION OF FOOD ENERGY

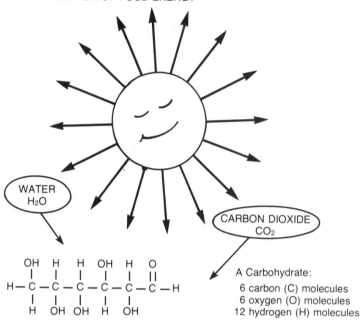

A Carbohydrate:

6 carbon (C) molecules
6 oxygen (O) molecules
12 hydrogen (H) molecules

II. CELLULAR METABOLISM: CONVERSION INTO USABLE ENERGY (ATP)

ADENOSINE TRIPHOSPHATE (ATP)

FIGURE 5.1 The process of energy conversion: The sun bonds together carbon, hydrogen, and oxygen molecules, storing this energy in our foods. Inside the cells of our body, foods are broken down and this stored energy is ultimately converted into the only energy source that the cell can utilize—adenosine triphosphate (ATP).

that transform food energy into ATP: aerobic oxidative and anaerobic glycolytic. These are not the only sources of the ATP utilized in exercise, but the others are extremely limited in comparison and are requried only by very specific muscular activities. Therefore we will discuss in detail only the aerobic-oxidative and anaerobic-glycolytic sources. The term *aerobic* means "with oxygen"; thus *anaerobic* is translated to mean "without oxygen." This categorization provides the basic precept for understanding of exercise prescription in terms of the energy requirement. Most fitness activities require energy from the aerobic-oxidative source, for the optimal stressing of the body's oxygen-transport system (see Chapter 6 for details), which delivers oxygen to the exercising muscles, is their most important physiological objective. In turn, this restricts the type and intensity of the activities that can be prescribed.

1. The Demand for ATP During Muscular Exercise

The concentration of ATP in a muscle cell is analogous to the high-water level in a reservoir: if the water behind the dam is to maintain an energy potential, its level must remain high at all times, even when the floodgate at the base of the dam is opened wide (see Figure 5.2). Similarly, the normal concentration of ATP in a muscle cell must be maintained even during the extreme demands of exercise. If the concentration of ATP in a muscle cell declines by approximately 40 percent—which can occur rapidly during very intense exercise—the muscular effort will either cease or at the very least will be severely impaired[1]. When exercise commences, the floodgates of the dam are suddenly opened, so to speak. Thus the principal role of the energy sources is to replenish cellular ATP at a rate corresponding to its utilization, and thereby to maintain a constant concentration of it in each muscle cell. During exercises of mild to moderate intensity, replenishment of ATP is easily accomplished by the energy sources, since the muscle's demand for ATP is well within their energy-generating capacities. As exercise intensifies, however, these capacities progressively diminish. In very strenuous exercise, the demand for ATP within the working muscle can increase more than fifteenfold. Consequently, the concentration of ATP within the muscle cell—and thus its immediate availability to the actin and myosin—can fall precipitously, and this will eventually result in cessation of the muscular effort. This is probably what occurs in weight lifting: after only a few repetitions (5 to 10 seconds) the weight lifter is unable to perform another repetition. During this very brief period of intense exercise ATP was being rapidly generated, but was insufficient because of the extreme energy demands created by repeated lifting of the heavy weight. Subjectively, this can be observed: after completing 5 to 10 seconds of pressing an extremely heavy weight with the leg muscles, weight lifters can immediately engage in less intense activities—walking, jogging, even mild to moderate running—as long as their energy demands are now within the energy-generating capacities of the intramuscular sources.

2. The Anaerobic-Glycolytic Energy Source

The anaerobic-glycolytic source is a system of complex and specialized enzymes that metabolize only carbohydrate molecules. The products of glycolysis (see Figure 5.2) are energy, in the form of ATP, heat, and lactic acid, perhaps the most maligned biochemical in the folklore of exercise physiology and sports training. (At this point, let it suffice to note that lactic acid is produced from

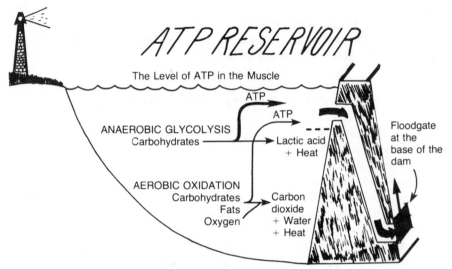

FIGURE 5.2 The ATP "reservoir" in muscle: A relatively high concentration of ATP must be maintained in the muscle in order for exercise to continue. The extent to which the "floodgate" is raised is analogous to the energy demanded by the exercise. During physical activity the intramuscular energy sources attempt to replenish ATP at the rate it is being expended; during heavy exercise this becomes impossible and the level of ATP in the muscle cell declines precipitously.

the breakdown of carbohydrates in the muscles during heavy exercise; however, its physiological effects are minimal compared with the vital role that the anaerobic-glycolytic source must play during intense exercise.) Anaerobic glycolysis is capable of generating a relatively large volume of ATP very rapidly, and without this energy source our capacity for exercise, particularly speed and power activities, would be severely limited. On the other hand, there are major disadvantages to performing exercises that require extensive amounts of energy from anaerobic glycolysis. In particular, this energy source has only a modest capacity for generating ATP over any sustained period: 45 to 70 seconds is the limit once *intense* muscular activity has commenced. Even though the expenditure of anaerobic-glycolytic energy will cause a concomitant elevation of the body's oxygen-transport system, this period of time is short and will always prove stressful to the individual.

3. The Aerobic-Oxidative Energy Source

The aerobic-oxidative source is an even more complex enzymatic pathway than glycolysis; it can metabolize both carbohydrates and fats. For the muscle to generate significant amounts of ATP from this source, however, an elevated level of oxygen is also required. During exercise, the aerobic generation of ATP is always in direct proportion to the volume of oxygen being consumed by the muscles. Consequently, the larger the volume of oxygen transported and consumed by the working muscles, the greater the volume of ATP generated. However, oxygen itself is not an energy source, as many mistakenly believe. Rather, it is a gas whose final disposition in the muscle cell is to chemically combine with two hydrogen atoms to form a molecule of water ($2H^+ + ½ O_2^- \rightarrow H_2O$). In addition to ATP and a small volume of water, the other end products of aerobic oxidation are carbon dioxide and, as in all exothermic reactions, heat. The volume of carbon dioxide produced in the muscle cell is approximately equal to the volume of oxygen consumed (see Figure 5.2).

Compared with anaerobic glycolysis, the aerobic-oxidative energy source is incapable of generating as much ATP over a similar time period, mainly because of its dependence upon the delivery of oxygen to the exercising muscle. However, when the intensity of the activity is such that aerobic oxidation can provide *all* of the ATP required by the muscles, there will be a number of important consequences for fitness:

1. The aerobic source can be utilized over a prolonged period of time—for example, 20 to 40 minutes for a jogger, and more than two hours for a marathon runner.
2. Over a prolonged period of exercise, there will be a sustained but healthful stimulus of the body's oxygen-transport system—a major goal of fitness prescription.
3. More of the body's stores of carbohydrates and fats will be metabolized as energy substrates.
4. The intensity of the activity will seldom prove too stressful, and after the initial 6 to 8 weeks of fitness prescription it can actually prove quite invigorating. In fact, the growth in popularity of fitness exercises and recreational activities over the past decade has been a direct result of this: correctly prescribed aerobic activities have proved beneficial without being overly stressful.

One final word before we conclude this section on the intramuscular source of ATP. More and more, muscle cells are being classified as either "red" or "white," "slow-twitch" or "fast-twitch," Type I or Type II—or even Type IIA, IIB, or IIC. These descriptive terms all call attention to the fact that groups of muscle cells with certain common characteristics (termed motor units) are better suited for one type of activity than another. Although every skeletal muscle cell possesses both glycolytic and oxidative enzymes, the point to appreciate is that all the muscle cells in a motor unit have a greater potential for generating ATP from one source than from the other, and thus are better suited to an activity of, say, endurance versus sustained speed versus power. Furthermore, each muscle cell possesses additional characteristics appropriate for the type of activity to which the motor unit is best suited. These facts have given rise to the profusion of terms used over the years in connection with muscle cell physiology. Thus muscle cells that have a superior aerobic-oxidative energy potential and are therefore better suited to rhythmic endurance activities have at various times been classified as *red, slow-twitch,* and *Type I.* On the other hand, muscle cells that possess fewer oxidative enzymes but a superior anaerobic-glycolytic potential and are thus better able to perform speed and power activities have been classified as *white, fast-twitch,* and *Type II.* These various characteristics of muscle types are summarized in Table 5.1.

THE ENERGY CONTINUUM: FROM REST
TO MAXIMAL EXERCISE

The intensity of exercise can be described qualitatively in several ways, such as: light, mild, half-speed maximal, exhausting, full-speed; and between these two extremes it can be subjectively gauged at any specific intensity. Exercise intensity can also be empirically quantified: according to the elevation of heart rate during exercise (see Chapter 8); through the rate of oxygen consumption; by the speed at which the person is walking, running, or cycling. In this section we will explain the energy continuum in both qualitative and quantitative terms. Since the energy that is generated at rest or in preexercise is much less than the energy required by supramaximal exercise, the important concepts in this section will be *when* the various intramuscular energy sources are utilized and *how* they are utilized in relation to the intensity of the exercise.

Why does the human machine possess two main intramuscular sources of energy plus additional small reservoirs of ATP within the muscles, when most

TABLE 5.1 Muscle Types and Characteristics

Earliest classification	Red	White	
Fiber type	Type I	Type II	
		A	B
Contraction characteristics	Slow-twitch	Fast-twitch	
Predominant energy source	Aerobic	Glycolytic	
Predominant activity	Rhythmic/ Endurance	Speed/Power	

machines require only a single energy source? The automobile, for example, has a combustion engine. The energy output from this single source is always in direct proportion to the rate of combustion, and whatever the rate of energy generated, it can be maintained over long periods. Applying this analogy to the human "engine" exercising, no single energy source within muscle possesses the same relative power or capacity of the combustion engine. At rest and through mild to moderate exercise, the aerobic source has both the power and the capacity, albeit low, to supply all of the muscles' energy requirements. However as exercise intensifies further, the aerobic source and its support systems become incapable of supplying all of the energy required[2]. Thus the anaerobic-glycolytic source must begin to supplement the relatively large volume of ATP already being generated by the aerobic source. For most healthy individuals, this occurs at about 50 to 66 percent of their maximal working capacity—or, more simply, when they begin to run faster than half-speed. The point at which glycolytic supplementation begins is referred to as the *anaerobic threshold*. In the more physically fit person this threshold occurs at a higher percentage of maximal working capacity—that is, closer to 66 percent (see Figure 5.3).

Very strenuous exercise results in the greatest demand for energy supplementation from anaerobic glycolysis. This exercise intensity cannot be continued indefinitely because of the limits of the glycolytic energy source. If the energy requirements of very heavy exercise cannot be met by the large contributions from the aerobic source plus major supplementation from glycolysis (as we have seen, 45 to 70 seconds of maximal demand will deplete the energy generated by glycolysis), exhaustion will occur. The reasons for this physiological state are not clearly understood, but at the point of exhaustion two consequences invariably occur: first, nonspecific yet subjectively noxious stimuli appear; second, the intensity of the exercise must be immediately reduced. On the other hand, exercise need not cease at the point of exhaustion; its intensity need only be reduced to the point where the aerobic source can supply all of the required energy.

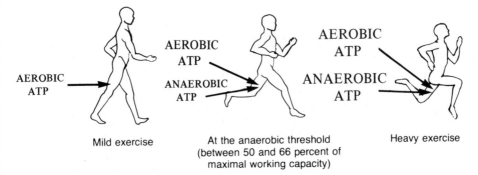

Mild exercise   At the anaerobic threshold   Heavy exercise
(between 50 and 66 percent of
maximal working capacity)

FIGURE 5.3 Energy contributions for the aerobic and anaerobic sources during exercise of varying intensities: walking, running just over half-speed, and sprinting.

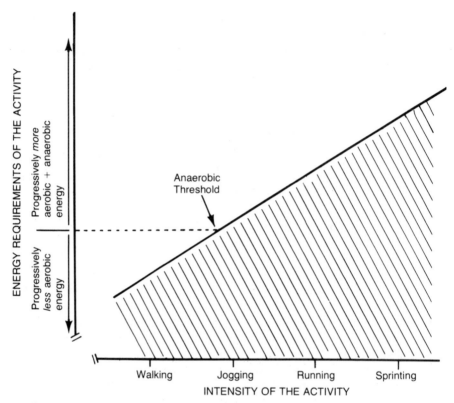

FIGURE 5.4 The energy continuum: the generation of ATP by the aerobic source only (below the anerobic threshold) and by the aerobic and anaerobic sources (above the anaerobic threshold) in relation to the intensity of the activity. The anaerobic threshold is attained between 50 and 66 percent of maximal (100 percent) exercise intensity.

Throughout the energy continuum, from very light to maximal exercise, progressively more oxygen must be delivered to the working muscles if they are to obtain increasing amounts of ATP from the aerobic-oxidative source. Above the anaerobic threshold particularly, energy production by the aerobic source becomes greatly elevated, but always in direct relation to the intensity of the exercise, up to its maximal capacity. Therefore exercise intensity (the x-axis in Figure 5.4) can be precisely quantified in terms of the volume of oxygen (in liters per minute) being delivered to the exercising muscle (see Table 5.2). Similarly, the elevation of the body's oxygen-transport system (the y-axis in Figure 5.4) can be precisely quantified in terms of any of several physiological parameters, heart rate (in beats per minute) being the most common. Therefore, the descriptive terms used in Figure 5.4 can be replaced by precise quantitative axes (see Figure 5.5).

TABLE 5.2 Average Oxygen-Consumption Values for Males and Females Performing Mild through Maximal Exercise

EXERCISE INTENSITY		OXYGEN CONSUMPTION (liters per minute)	
Description	Effort	x̄ Values for Males	x̄ Values for Females
Maximal	100%	4.0	3.5
Heavy	66–90%	2.7–3.6	2.3–3.2
Moderate	50%	2.0	1.7
Mild	25–40%	1.0–1.6	0.8–1.5
Rest/Preexercise	<10%	0.4	0.3

It should now be obvious why lower-intensity, endurance activities prove much more beneficial to fitness: they require more aerobic and less anaerobic energy, they place a healthful stress on the body's physiological support systems, yet they utilize more energy because they can be carried out over a longer period. For optimal fitness benefits to accrue, however, what should the specific exercise intensity be for a given individual? How long should the activity be carried out during an exercise session? How many times per week should this stress be imposed? These are critical considerations, for too low an exercise intensity for a particular individual can prove ineffectual whereas too great an intensity can prove noxious, even harmful. And of course no two persons are exactly alike.

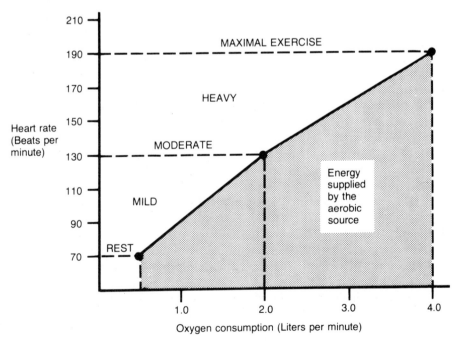

FIGURE 5.5 The aerobic-energy continuum: the intensity of exercise, from mild through maximal, as measured by the oxygen consumed and the directly proportionate increase in heart rate.

THE PHYSIOLOGY OF RECOVERY FROM EXERCISE

Another important component of exercise prescription and one that is often ignored by the novice is a proper "cool-down" following the activity. Most people are aware of the importance of a warm-up—a short period in which the intensity of exercise is gradually increased—and most feel the need for it (see Chapter 8). Likewise, the strenuous component in an exercise session should never end abruptly, but rather should be followed by appropriate light activity (see Chapter 8). Just as the body must be adequately warmed up prior to exercise, it should be carefully cooled down afterwards. This necessitates a basic understanding of the physiology of recovery, perhaps the most misunderstood aspect of exercise physiology.

After 30 to 40 minutes of mild exercise (warm-up and flexibility exercises) and then relatively strenuous exercise (the main portion of the exercise prescription), approximately 1 to 2 hours are required to return the body to its preexercise homeostatic (normal resting) state. The time for recovery varies with four factors: the intensity and the duration of the activity; the environmental conditions (temperature, humidity, and so forth); and in particular the fitness of the participant. The fitter individual recovers more quickly than the unfit person following similar amounts of activity. A person who is still fatigued an hour or so following a workout has probably undertaken too much exercise for his or her fitness level. Exercise directly involves, or indirectly affects, almost all of the neural, hormonal, biochemical, and other physiological systems of the body. Thus recovery from exercise must be a highly complex process as well. *Recovery,* then, is the physiological term for the myriad processes that return the body from its elevated state following the healthful stress of exercise to its normal resting metabolic state and function. Though a complex physiological process, it occurs efficiently and completely following correctly prescribed exercise. Recovery requires energy, and this energy is obtained exclusively from the aerobic source. Therefore, it is only reasonable that oxygen consumption should remain elevated following cessation of exercise and remain so for some time thereafter (see Figure 5.6).

In the 1920s this continued elevation of oxygen consumption in recovery was called the *oxygen debt,* but this term conveyed the erroneous impression that oxygen had been borrowed from somewhere during the exercise. Later research confirmed that the body has no "oxygen vaults" and stores an extremely limited amount of oxygen (only 1 or 2 liters, which are contained in the lungs and dissolved throughout the body). Curiously, *oxygen debt* has recently become synonymous with anaerobic metabolism, the presence of lactic acid in the body following strenuous exercise, and almost exclusively with only short-term, very intense exercise. Though a complex physiological process, the level of lactic acid in the body can be quite elevated following a strenuous exercise session, as are body temperature, the endocrine responses, the cardiorespiratory systems, and many other physiological functions. The approximate time for these functions

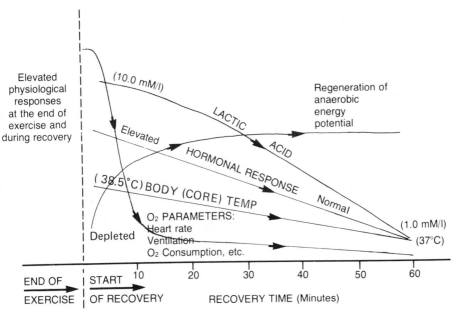

Elevated
physiological
responses
at the end of
exercise and
during recovery

(10.0 mM/l)

LACTIC ACID

Regeneration of
anaerobic
energy
potential

Elevated

HORMONAL RESPONSE

Normal

(38.5°C) BODY (CORE) TEMP

(1.0 mM/l)

(37°C)

Depleted

O₂ PARAMETERS:
Heart rate
Ventilation
O₂ Consumption, etc.

END OF
EXERCISE

START
OF RECOVERY

10   20   30   40   50   60

RECOVERY TIME (Minutes)

FIGURE 5.6   Recovery: the period in which the physiological systems of the body
are returned to their normal preexercise levels.

to return to their normal levels is illustrated in Figure 5.6. When a large amount
of lactic acid has been produced during exercise, it is metabolized steadily but
slowly over the recovery period[3].

A cool-down period can assist the recovery process, particularly during
the first 10 minutes after exercise, when the internal physiological functions are
most elevated. A proper cool-down bridges the gap between the exercise session
and complete cessation of activity, and can greatly assist the circulatory system
in its return to a normal metabolic level. Stretching the muscles after exercise
has been shown to reduce the stiffness one may experience the day after the
workout. It is inadvisable to consume a cold beverage or take an extremely
warm shower immediately afterwards. Only small sips of cold water should be
taken during the 10-minute cool-down.

APPLICATION OF THE ENERGY CONTINUUM: CONTINUOUS
VERSUS INTERMITTENT EXERCISE

Why has jogging gained such widespread popularity? For one thing, everyone
has the skill to participate, for jogging is one of the simplest motor skills. Second,
facilities are available to everyone—the great outdoors if indoor facilities are
nonexistent. Most important, continuous, submaximal activity below the anaerobic threshold can prove enjoyable and provide an almost universal recipe
for attaining fitness. However, a large percentage of those who are concerned

about their fitness intensely dislike the boredom they find inherent in jogging, or else they live in the center of a city, where facilities for jogging are restricted, or they simply prefer the challenge of more complex sports skills and the venue of competition. Whatever the reasons, these persons may select a popular sports activity as the major component of their exercise program (see Chapter 9).

1. Continuous Exercise: A Specific Exercise Intensity Maintained Over Time

The physiological response to muscular activity can vary greatly. This is particularly evident in the energy requirements for single bouts of specific activities, each carried out over a certain period. Consider the activities presented in Figure 5.7: lifting a heavy weight for 4 seconds, sprinting for 11 seconds (100 meters), sprinting for 60 seconds (400 meters, but at a slightly reduced speed), and jogging for 30 minutes at an oxygen-consumption rate of 1.5 to 1.8 liters per minute (in other words, at approximately 40-percent of maximum intensity). The energy requirements for each activity are unique, but there are some common elements that can help us understand the universal application of the energy continuum in all four cases. Note that the aerobic-energy contribution at the onset of each activity is minimal. Thereafter, time is required in order for the aerobic contribution to significantly increase. However, neither 4 seconds of weight lifting nor 11 seconds of sprinting is sufficient to significantly increase the aerobic contributions to these exercises, even though their intensity is high. Usually up to one minute of exercise is required before the oxygen-transport system begins to deliver a substantial volume of oxygen to the working muscles (see activities on the right in Figure 5.7)[4].

On the other hand, in each of the examples in Figure 5.7 the anaerobic energy, immediately and readily available in the working-muscle cells, makes up the difference between the energy available at any one time from the aerobic source and the total energy requirement for the activity. For example, in 4 seconds of weight lifting, the aerobic contribution is extremely small yet the intensity of this exercise requires the greatest and most immediate demand for ATP; this difference can be supplied only by anaerobic energy. In contrast, jogging requires only a very minor anaerobic contribution, for the ATP required throughout this activity is well within the capacities of the aerobic energy source. Finally, in any exercise surpassing the anaerobic threshold, anaerobic energy must be utilized, and in ever-increasing amounts as the exercise intensifies.

2. Intermittent Exercise: Exercise Whose Intensity Constantly Varies

Activities and sports played at high exercise intensities must employ intermittent activity. That is, relief periods—short intervals of less intense activity

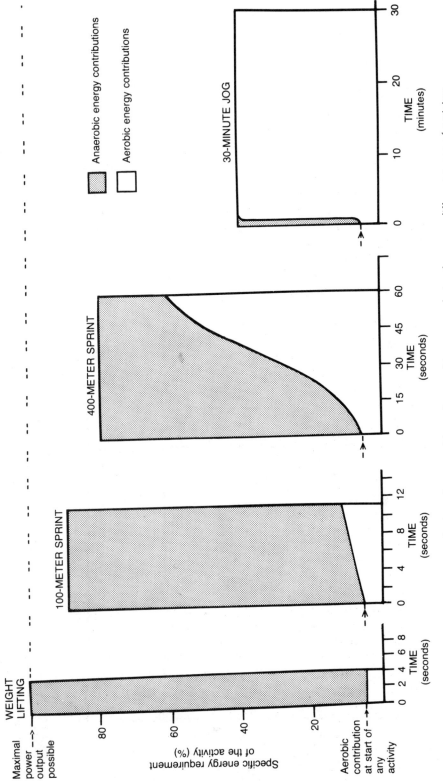

FIGURE 5.7 The energy contributions from aerobic and anaerobic sources during four very different types of activites.

57

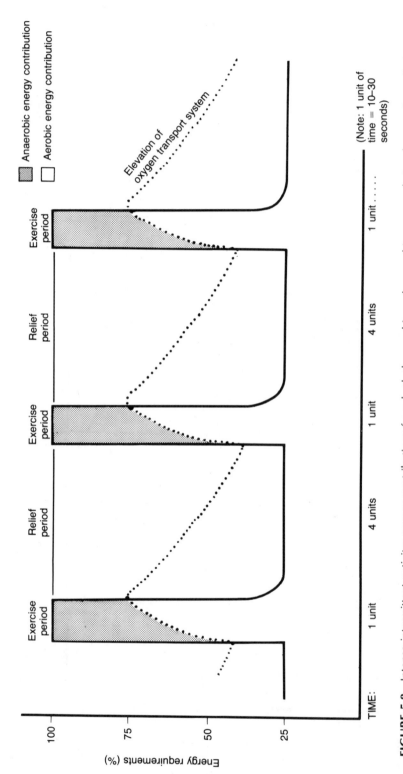

FIGURE 5.8 Intense intermittent activity: energy contributions from both the aerobic and anaerobic sources during the exercise periods (very high intensity), and from the aerobic source only during the relief periods (intensity greatly reduced, no anaerobic energy required). Note that the oxygen-transport system, elevated in each exercise period, begins to recover during the subsequent relief periods. The time ratio of exercise to relief period is 1 to 4.

(activity below the anaerobic threshold)—must be interspersed among the phases of intense exercise. In fact, intermittent activity characterizes the vast majority of popular North American activities and sports—all the racquet sports, basketball, hockey, football, soccer, and so on. In intermittent exercise, as in continuous exercise, aerobic-energy generation begins to accelerate at the commencement of intense exercise and will become elevated in direct proportion to the intensity of the activity if it is of sufficient duration; at the end of a period of intense activity the oxygen-transport system begins to recover (slow down). On the other hand, anaerobic energy will always supplement the aerobic contributions to the extent required and for as long as each short phase of intense activity is maintained (see Figure 5.8).

There are two important cautions that one should appreciate if recreational sports activities are to provide the healthful stress and enjoyable experience intended by exercise prescription.

a. Length of the Exercise Period. Over a prolonged exercise period—for example, an extended volley in tennis or squash—the drain on anaerobic energy can be considerable. Over a series of such periods, even when interspersed with lengthy relief periods, the anaerobic-energy drain can have a profound cumulative effect. The participant will feel fatigued and his or her level of skill will deteriorate. Therefore, the length of the average exercise period throughout a game or competition is a compromise relative to the intensity of the activity. The more intense the activity during the exercise period, the greater the anaerobic-energy utilization per second, and thus the shorter the length of each exercise period must be (less than 5 seconds in very intense exercise) or else the resulting fatigue will prove too stressful.

b. Length of the Relief Period. In intermittent activity, relief periods must be neither too short nor inordinately long. Each must be sufficiently long to ensure that some of the anaerobic potential expended during the previous exercise period is restored[5]. However, it cannot be too long, for it will then give the oxygen-transport system too much time to recover.

The rule of thumb for achieving optimal fitness benefits and enjoyment from sports activities while minimizing the physical stress on the participant is an exercise-to-relief ratio of one to three. For example, if each exercise period consists of 10 seconds of intense activity, the relief periods should be (about) 30 seconds. As a corollary to this general principle, the less intense the activity, the longer each exercise period (and the shorter each relief period) may be. However, the exercise-to-relief ratio should seldom decline below one to two.

SPORTS TRAINING VERSUS FITNESS PRESCRIPTION

Intermittent activity employing intense to maximal exercise interspersed with only short relief periods should never be confused with fitness prescription. The former is more correctly termed *interval training*, and is used in competitive sports. The folklore of physical training contains an old adage that far too many fitness enthusiasts still believe: no pain, no gain. This also has little relevance to fitness prescription. Pain and excess fatigue during workout mean that anaerobic glycolysis has become a major contributor of ATP for the activity. In fitness prescription, the utilization of anaerobic energy should be moderate at best, and only then in enjoyable competitive situations. Stated another way, physical exertion must be positive rather than noxious if it is to be incorporated into one's lifestyle.

On the other hand, the competitive athlete must learn to live with pain, since most athletic events, whether intermittent or continuous, are performed at high intensities and therefore require substantial anaerobic glycolysis. The intensity and duration of training exercises are set according to the requirements of the sport, as is the complexity of their motor skills. Thus, training methods that mimic competitive conditions are prerequisites for participation in a competitive sport, and the athlete must willingly accept any excesses or abuses that they contain. Moreover, an athlete's training must be geared to developing specific energy capacities and complex neuromuscular skills.

Another widespread misconception regarding sports training is that a highly skilled athlete is in shape for a wide range of athletic endeavors. Nothing could be further from the truth! Contrast the component skills in basketball, football, gymnastics, tennis, and so on. Note the different physical proportions of athletes in different sports, and even the range of physical characteristics among athletes in the same sport (football, for example). Important differences among the energy capacities of athletes in various sports and, more important, the effect of their specific training regimens can then be appreciated. Sports training is highly utilitarian, participation usually involves very intense and uniquely specific training, and highly competitive sports require substantial anaerobic-glycolytic energy.

The concept and the goals of exercise prescription are much different. However, since many exercise and sports activities overlap, there is confusion between sports training and fitness. First and foremost, exercise prescription is not training and should never be considered as such. Training uses activities and exercises, regardless of how painful or excessive, to achieve a competitive goal: winning through athletic excellence. Exercise prescription, on the other hand, embodies physical effort that is positive, pleasurable, even exhilarating; in fact, only in this way can fitness enthusiasts hope to continue a physical activity throughout their lifetime.

Second, sports training is intrinsically involved with intramuscular energy production and therefore the development of the hereditary aerobic and anaerobic potential that athletes must bring to their sport[6]. Exercise prescription places demands on the aerobic source that are well within an individual's maximal capacities. This stimulus is never intended to train this intramuscular source per se. Rather, it is a means for effecting a healthful stress on the lungs, heart, and vascular system.

Third, the skill components in competitive sports have become highly specialized. However, in fitness activities specific skills are of minor importance, except, of course, among fitness enthusiasts who select a sport as their activity and compete against friends with similar skill levels.

Finally, whereas the reasons for competitive-sports participation are very narrow, a wide range of personal factors influence the individual's participation in fitness activities. Enhancing general health and vigor, reducing body mass, and promoting a sense of well-being may be the specific objectives of one's program. In addition, physical criteria such as sex, age, and health (discussed in Chapters 8 and 9) must modify one's prescription. The locale, the available facilities, and one's previous sports or activity experiences will also influence participation in an exercise program. And there is no doubt that each of the many people who engage in fitness could add another personal reason for his or her participation.

REFERENCES

1. J. Bergstrom, R. C. Harris, E. Hultman and L. O. Nordesjo, "Energy Rich Phosphogens in Dynamic and Static Work," in *Advances in Experimental Medicine and Biology, Vol. 11, Muscle Metabolism During Exercise,* ed. Bengt Pernow and Bengt Saltin (New York: Plenum, 1971), pp. 341–55.

2. J. Karlsson, "Muscle ATP, CP, and Lactate in Submaximal and Maximal Exercise," in *Muscle Metabolism During Exercise,* pp. 383–93.

3. A. N. Belcastro and A. Bonen, "Lactic Acid Removal Rates During Controlled and Uncontrolled Recovery Exercise," *Journal of Applied Physiology,* 39 (1975), 932–36.

4. J. M. Thomson and K. J. Garvie, "A Laboratory Method for Determination of Anaerobic Energy Expenditure During Sprinting," *Canadian Journal of Applied Sports Sciences,* 6 (1981), 21–26.

5. B. Saltin and B. Essen, "Muscle Glycogen, Lactate, ATP, and CP in Intermittent Exercise," in *Muscle Metabolism During Exercise,* ed. Pernow and Saltin, pp. 419–24.

6. D. L. Costill, J. Daniels, W. Evans, W. Fink, G. Krahenbuhl, and B. Saltin, "Skeletal Muscle Enzymes and Fiber Composition in Male and Female Track Athletes," *Journal of Applied Physiology,* 40 (1976), 149–54.

6

The Physiological Systems: Support for Muscle Activity

INTRODUCTION

Muscular exercise requires the simultaneous operation of many support systems in the body—some critically important for the performance of the activity, others less important. In competitive sports, the operation of these physiological systems are of secondary concern; successful performance is the ultimate goal. In exercise prescription the opposite holds true: the stimulus placed upon the many physiological systems that support the contraction of the muscles provides the primary motive for the activity. Stated another way, placing an optimal stress on specific body systems through healthful exercise should be a major goal of fitness prescription; how skillfully one performs whatever mode of activity has been chosen is far less important. In addition, this activity must satisfy the needs of the participant, for each individual has different physiological capacities, needs, and goals.

In this chapter we describe the physiological reactions that are important to the exercise prescriptionist. The most important support system is the oxygen-transport system because of its involvement in energy generation within the muscles. As we saw in the last chapter, the rate at which this system operates is always in direct response to the intensity of the exercise stimulus. Another physiological function that is related very closely to the intensity of the activity, particularly if it consists of 30 minutes to an hour of vigorous exercise, is the temperature-regulating mechanism of the body, which has immediate consequences on both the comfort and safety of the participant. Diet and nutrition provide another important support for exercise, and the percentage of one's body fat has a particularly significant bearing on fitness. Many physiological functions, while not directly supporting muscular activity, are vital to the daily maintenance of the body and therefore the general health and vigor of the individual. At the end of the chapter we discuss some other factors in exercise prescription: gender, heredity, aging, and lifestyle factors such as stress, tobacco, and alcohol.

THE OXYGEN–TRANSPORT SYSTEM

The body possesses a highly integrated system for extracting oxygen from the air and transporting it to the cells. The same process continuously brings carbon dioxide from the cells to the lungs, where it is expired (see Figure 6.1)[1]. In this section we detail the two main components of the oxygen-transport system: the *respiratory system,* which comprises the lungs and pulmonary circulation, and the *cardiovascular system,* which includes the heart and systemic circulation—the vast vascular network that channels blood to every cell in the body.

A great deal has been researched and written about the oxygen-transport system, yet its basic function and physiology are still not widely understood. The respiratory system serves one vital purpose: by means of a pair of unique organs, the lungs, it facilitates the gas exchange between body and atmosphere that oxygenates the blood. The cardiovascular system distributes this oxygenated blood to the cells of the body; during exercise much of the oxygenated blood is channeled directly to the working muscles. The cardiovascular system has many other physiological functions to perform since it is the main delivery system for the body. It transports nutrients, water, and various chemicals, including hormones, and carries away the by-products of cellular metabolism, including carbon dioxide and heat. Some of these functions are of direct concern to the exercise prescriptionist and will be discussed in this section.

The oxygen-transport system must always be operating; if not, life will terminate in 4 to 6 minutes. Yet the constant low level of operation of the system is not sufficient to maintain its functional excellence[2]. Aging, heredity, and particularly lifestyle factors such as job-related pressures and smoking can all reduce its level of excellence. The incidence of respiratory, heart, and vascular diseases in North America is staggering; the annual health-care costs alone for these diseases amount to billions of dollars. On the other hand, properly prescribed exercise imposes a healthful overload on the oxygen-transport system, forcing it to regularly function at an elevated rate for a limited period of time. Such a periodic stress has been shown to both retard the functional decline of the system and improve its operational excellence. Correctly prescribed exercise will produce significant improvements in function and capacity within 6 to 10 weeks; subjectively, maintaining these improvements thereafter will seem to require even less effort.

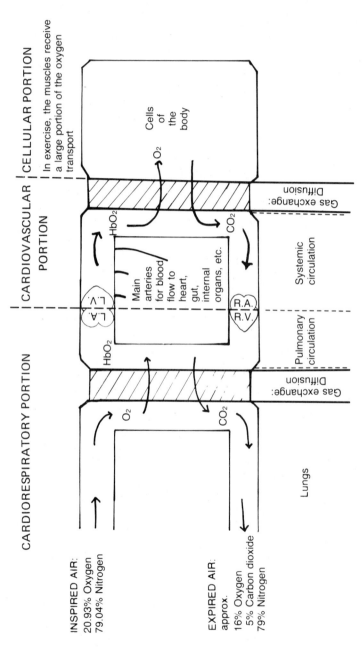

FIGURE 6.1 Oxygen-transport system. Air, which contains 20.93% oxygen (O_2), enters the lungs. A small amount of this O_2 diffuses into the blood, where it combines chemically with hemoglobin (HbO_2). The circulatory system, by means of its main pumping station, the left side of the heart—the left atrium (L.A.) and left ventricle (L.V.)—distributes the blood to every cell in the body. Some of the O_2 (as much as is needed) diffuses from the blood into the cells. The system for transport of carbon dioxide from the cells to the lungs is almost the reverse of this process, and is assisted by the right side of the heart—the right atrium (R.A.) and right ventricle (R.V.). *Source:* Adapted from Alf Holmgren and Per-Olof Åstrand, "D_L and the Dimensions and Functional Capacities of the O_2 Transport System in Humans," *Journal of Applied Physiology,* 21 (1966), 1465. Used by permission.

The Respiratory System: Exercise Ventilation
for Gas Exchange

Contraction of the diaphragm, intercostal, and other respiratory muscles creates a partial vacuum in the lungs. As a result, air is inspired through the nasal passages and mouth and then distributed to the approximately 3 billion terminal air sacs (*alveoli*) in the lung (see Figure 6.2). Expiration is the reverse of this process: relaxation of the diaphragm and intercostal muscles causes a

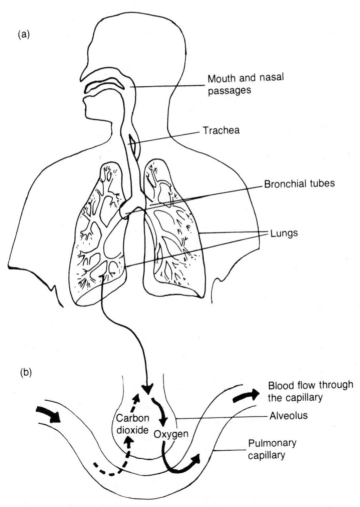

FIGURE 6.2   The respiratory system: (a) air-conduction network in the lungs; (b) gas exchange, in an alvelous (terminal air sac), between air and blood.

buildup of air pressure in the lungs that forces alveolar air out. When more air must be expired more forcefully, as during exercise, coughing, or sneezing, contraction of the abdominal muscles assists in expiration. At rest, the amount of air we breathe is usually less than 10 liters per minute. However, with the commencement of physical activity both the depth of each breath (the *tidal volume*) and the number of breaths each minute rapidly increase. A healthy adult engaged in heavy exercise can ventilate over 100 liters of air per minute. The volume of air that must be taken into the lungs each. minute—*exercise ventilation*—is illustrated in Figure 6.3.

Two important aspects of exercise ventilation are not fully understood or appreciated. First, the air in our environment consists of only 20.93 percent oxygen (by volume); the remainder is almost entirely nitrogen (79.04 percent). During gas exchange in the lungs, however, nitrogen is physiologically inert. Therefore four-fifths of the tidal volume serves no physiological purpose! In heavy exercise, when one is breathing 100 liters of air per minute, the effort required to inspire, then expire, 80 liters of nitrogen can become very burdensome. Second, our ventilatory efforts are wasted even further in that only a small portion of the oxygen we inspire becomes involved in gas exchange. We inspire air that is 20.93 percent oxygen, yet our expired air is approximately 16 percent oxygen. (This abundance of oxygen in our expired air explains why mouth-to-mouth resuscitation can be so effective in saving lives.) If we combine these two facts, we find that about 95 percent of the air we breathe at rest or during exercise is merely inspired, mixed with the air already in the alveoli (where it raises the concentration of oxygen slightly), and then expired. The result is that during exercise, when the working muscles demand much more oxygen, the volume of air that we rhythmically inspire, then expire, must increase by a factor of *at least* 20 times.

While ventilation is being carried on continuously by the lungs, venous blood is constantly being pumped from the right ventricle of the heart through the pulmonary artery and then dispersed into the small capillaries that surround the alveoli (Figure 6.4). In a person at rest, the oxygen content of the venous blood returning to the lungs is depleted by up to 25 percent. However, even in light to moderate exercise up to 85 percent of the blood's oxygen can be depleted[3]. At the same time, the level of carbon dioxide in the venous blood has increased relative to the body's rate of metabolism. Thus as venous blood enters a pulmonary capillary immediately adjacent to a well-ventilated alveolus, oxygen diffuses from the alveolus into the blood while carbon dioxide diffuses in the opposite direction. The blood that leaves the pulmonary capillary has therefore been *arterialized*—its oxygen content has been replenished and its carbon dioxide diminished.

In order for gas diffusion to occur, the tissues of the lungs must be thin and delicate. In comparison, a sheet of very thin tissue paper would be almost like a layer of steel. This explains why smoking, inhaled drugs, and air pollutants are potentially so dangerous to the lungs. Exercise requires a great increase not

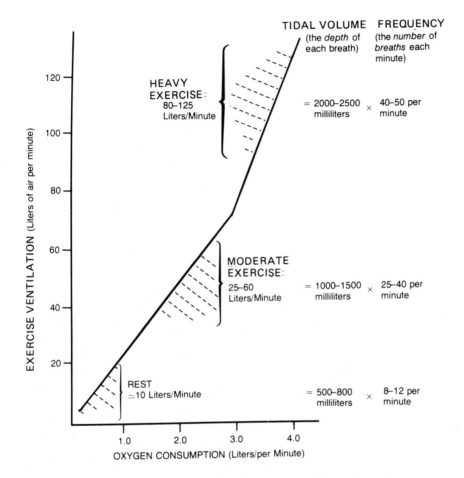

FIGURE 6.3 Exercise ventilation relative to exercise intensity. Exercise ventilation is the product of the depth of each breath (tidal volume) and the number of breaths per minute (frequency). Volume and frequency increase with the intensity of the exercise, but the specific combinations of the two are unique for each individual.

only in ventilation but in the volume of blood channeled to the lungs—up to a sixfold increase in very heavy exercise. However, from rest through maximal exercise the *healthy* respiratory system always performs its function perfectly; that is, arterialized blood is always almost 100 percent oxygenated to its capacity as it leaves the lungs[4]. On the other hand, as a gas exchanger the unhealthy lung can quickly become a disaster, even in mild exercise. Any impairment of one process—ventilation of the alveoli, perfusion of the capillaries with blood, or gas diffusion—results in an exponential problem within the system, since gas exchange cannot proceed unless all three processes function in unison.

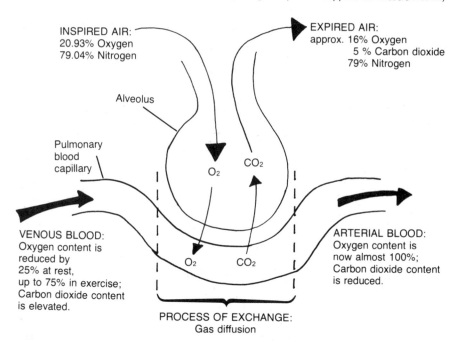

INSPIRED AIR:
20.93% Oxygen
79.04% Nitrogen

EXPIRED AIR:
approx. 16% Oxygen
        5 % Carbon dioxide
       79% Nitrogen

Alveolus

Pulmonary
blood
capillary

CO_2

O_2

VENOUS BLOOD:
Oxygen content is
reduced by
25% at rest,
up to 75% in exercise;
Carbon dioxide content
is elevated.

ARTERIAL BLOOD:
Oxygen content is
now almost 100%;
Carbon dioxide content
is reduced.

O_2 CO_2

PROCESS OF EXCHANGE:
Gas diffusion

FIGURE 6.4   Gas exchange is carried on continuously in the alveoli. With each breath the inspired air replenishes the oxygen in the alveolus; thus the venous blood being pumped to the lungs is constantly being arterialized in the pulmonary capillaries.

The benefits of regular fitness activity for the respiratory system can prove substantial, provided the system is free from clinical symptoms of disease. This should be determined by a physician prior to exercise prescription. In the healthy individual, exercise prescription will improve gas exchange very little, since it already functions perfectly in the healthy lung. However, exercise prescription will enhance both pulmonary circulation, particularly in the heart (see the next section in this chapter), and exercise ventilation. The latter improvement is one of the most noticeable during the initial 6 to 10 weeks of exercise. Ventilatory efforts are progressively reduced, tidal volume (the depth of breathing) increases, and the number of breaths per minute decreases. Moreover, since approximately 95 percent of the volume of air that we ventilate actually serves a nonphysiologic purpose, the amount of overventilation is progressively reduced[5]. One final word to conclude this section on the respiratory system. Many myths have been perpetuated regarding nonphysiological "miracles" (for lack of a better term) attributed to such practices as deep-breathing, the expelling of "bad vapors" from the body, the controlled breathing practiced by Eastern mystics, and so on. The scientific substance of these practices has not been substantiated by modern experimentation. Breathing can be controlled voluntarily, and deep breathing or controlled breathing may prove relaxing to some. In the final analysis, however, during exercise we *must breathe* in direct proportion to our metabolic needs, since oxygen is required by the muscles and oxygenation of the blood is one of the critical links in the oxygen transport system. Correctly prescribed exercise, if performed with regularity, is the most beneficial way to meet this requirement.

The Cardiovascular System: Oxygen Delivery to the Muscles during Exercise

The Heart. The cardiovascular portion of the oxygen transport system begins at the left ventricle of the heart, which receives the arterialized blood that returns from the lungs through the pulmonary vein into the left atrium of the heart (Figure 6.5). The left ventricle is referred to as the main pumping station of the body, but this title flatters the engineering shortcomings of the cardiovascular system. The left ventricle is a small chamber surrounded by muscular walls. When filled with blood, it is about the size of a clenched fist. With each muscular contraction of the heart, initiated by a self-generated electrical impulse (Figure 6.6), some of the blood is squeezed out of the left ventricle into the *aorta*, the main artery of the systemic circulation. This volume of blood is called the *stroke volume*. As exercise intensity increases, the contractions of the left ventricle must become more forceful, resulting in a progressively greater stroke volume (Figure 6.7).

With each heartbeat, therefore, the ventricular musculature must pressurize the blood in order to forcefully eject the stroke volume into the aorta, and this is where the cardiovascular system's inherent engineering fallibility becomes apparent. This relatively small muscular pump has a monumental task: from the left ventricle the blood must travel through the systemic vasculature, a distance of over 20 kilometers; for every kilogram of excess body fat this distance increases approximately 3.5 kilometers. The heart must continue to pressurize the blood, and it does so 70 times per minute (at rest), a minimum of 4200 times per hour, 100,800 times per day, 3.6×10^7 times per year—2.32×10^9 heartbeats over a life span of 70 years. Unlike almost every other tissue in the body, the heart *dare* not stop functioning, even if its own tissue ruptures or its own blood supply (the coronary circulation) becomes impaired.

Even from this perspective, the enormity of the burden placed on the heart is difficult to fully appreciate. The shocking statistics on heart disease that are reported annually are perhaps more revealing. A number of coronary-risk factors, which appear almost inconsequential and certainly not risky, have been identified by the American Heart Association (Table 6.1): diet, the number of cigarettes smoked each day, and, to a lesser degree, daily consumption of alcohol, job-related pressures—even one's hereditary predisposition to heart disease. Three other potential coronary risks are the percentage of one's body mass that is fat, the cholesterol level in one's blood, and one's exercise habits. It would take an extreme excess of any of these risk factors to cause a health problem in any other region of the body. (The liver and lungs are the only exceptions: excessive

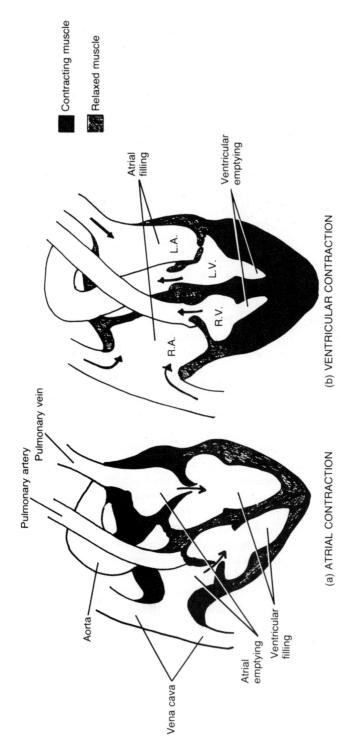

FIGURE 6.5 Phases of the four-chambered heart pump; (a) Blood from the right and left atria fills the ventricles; (b) blood from the right ventricle is pumped into the pulmonary artery, and blood from the left ventricle is pumped forcefully into the aorta, while the atria refill with blood.

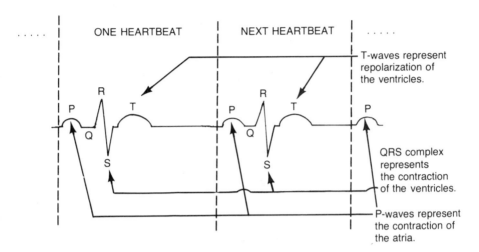

FIGURE 6.6 Electrocardiogram tracing: the sequencing of the heart's self-generated electrical activity, which initiates each phase of the heart's muscular contractions.

alcohol consumption and smoking, respectively, are specific risk factors for these organs.) Yet when the heart is at risk, even a minor excess of one factor can have dire consequences; the interactive effect of two or more risk factors exponentially increases one's chance of encountering coronary problems.

On the other hand, the healthy heart will perform its function magnificently and properly prescribed fitness exercise has repeatedly proved an important help to cardiac functioning[6]. Not only will correctly prescribed exercise maintain heart function, it can also improve it by slowing the rate (whether a lowered resting rate or a maximal rate) at which the heart must beat in response to any given level of metabolism. Regular exercise will also increase stroke volume and thereby maintain *cardiac output,* (the total blood flow, computed by multiplying heart rate by stroke volume). This can be accomplished with a reduction in the pressure that the left ventricle must impart to the blood. In contrast, sudden intense activity such as snow shoveling, an emergency, or a rare sports outing can prove extremely harmful if the health of the heart has been permitted to decline. However, fitness prescription alone is not a panacea, and therefore this textbook is as much a guide to a more healthful lifestyle as it is exercise prescription. The message is clear: our heart can use all the healthful assistance we can give it—every day, every year, for a lifetime.

The Vascular System. From the heart a vast tubular network distributes the arterialized blood to all parts of the body. Large-diameter tubes (the arteries) channel the blood into smaller tubes (arterioles), which in turn branch into a vast microscopic network (the capillary beds). A capillary lies adjacent to every cell in the body, permitting an exchange of oxygen and nutrients between it and

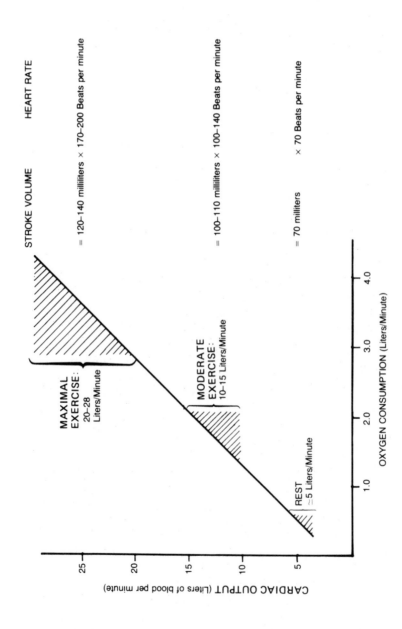

FIGURE 6.7 Relation of cardiac output (the volume of blood pumped out by the heart each minute) and exercise intensity. Stroke volume (the amount of blood squeezed by each heartbeat) multiplied by the heart rate (number of beats per minute) determines the cardiac output. Both stroke volume and heart rate increase in direct relation to the intensity of the exercise.

TABLE 6.1 Coronary Risk Factors Related to the Incidence of Heart Disease

PHYSIOLOGICAL FACTORS
1. Abnormal electrocardiogram
2. Elevated blood pressure
3. Excessive body fat
4. Elevated levels of blood lipids, primarily cholesterol
5. Heredity: family history of heart and vascular disease

LIFESTYLE FACTORS
6. Number of cigarettes smoked per day
7. Abnormal alcohol consumption
8. Job-related stress
9. Lack of regular physical activity or exercise

the blood. Other small-diameter tubes (venules) collect the blood leaving the capillaries, which then flows through larger and larger veins until it enters the right atrium of the heart through the inferior and superior venae cavae (Figure 6.8).

There is no beginning or end to this vascular system; it is a *circle* through which the blood circulates. However, for the blood to flow from the heart to the capillaries and back, the arterial side of the system must be highly pressurized, and this is why most heart and vascular problems arise (Figure 6.9). To ensure that each stroke volume will be pumped out of the left ventricle, the heart must exert pressure on the blood that is greater than the *diastolic* arterial blood pressure—that is, the existing pressure in the aorta and major arteries. In a healthy individual the diastolic pressure normally remains at about 80 mmHg,* both at rest and during exercise. As each stroke volume is squeezed out by the left ventricle, the pressure in the main arteries rapidly rises. This is termed *systolic* arterial blood pressure, and at rest it normally rises to a peak of 120 mmHg. However, during exercise the larger stroke volumes cause the systolic pressure to rise as high as 180 mmHg. Diastolic and systolic pressure is necessary for the normal functioning of the cardiovascular system, and the heart is well equipped to work against them. However, continual pressures higher than these normal values can chronically stress the heart. In persons with slight vascular problems, systolic pressure can exceed 220 mmHg during exercise, and this can be dangerous.

The pressure buildup in the arteries is minimized and dissipated by three mechanisms: (1) the size of the arterial cavity (*lumen*); (2) the elasticity of the arterial walls; and (3) the continual runoff of an equivalent volume of blood from the arteries into the vast network of capillary beds, which maintains a relatively constant volume of blood in the arterial network. Any alteration of these mechanisms can initiate a vicious circle: the ventricular musculature must

---

* Blood pressure is calculated in millimeter of mercury (mmHg).

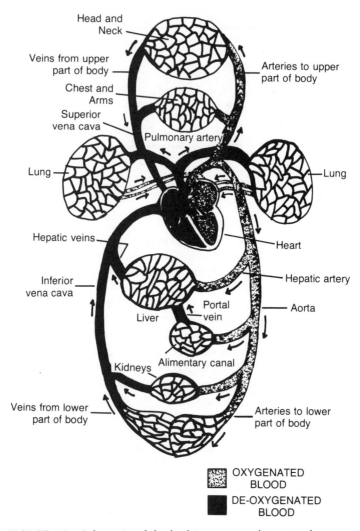

Head and Neck

Veins from upper part of body

Arteries to upper part of body

Chest and Arms

Superior vena cava

Pulmonary artery

Lung

Lung

Hepatic veins

Heart

Inferior vena cava

Hepatic artery

Portal vein

Liver

Aorta

Alimentary canal

Kidneys

Veins from lower part of body

Arteries to lower part of body

OXYGENATED BLOOD

DE-OXYGENATED BLOOD

FIGURE 6.8 Schematic of the body's vast vascular network. Arteries channel blood from the heart to every tissue and cell in the body; veins return the blood to the heart and lungs. *Source*: B.A. Schottelius and D.D. Schottelius, *Textbook of Physiology*, 18th ed. (St. Louis: The C.V. Mosby Co., 1978); reprinted by permission of the authors.

work harder and pressurize the blood substantially more; this elevates the pressure in the arteries, which in turn imposes an even greater workload on the heart.

A number of conditions have been shown to harm the basic health and integrity of the arteries. These conditions can lead eventually to hypertension (chronically high blood pressure). *Atherosclerosis* is a hardening of the artery

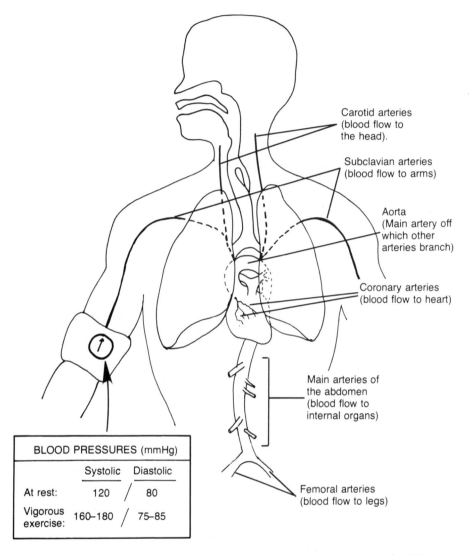

Carotid arteries
(blood flow to
the head).

Subclavian arteries
(blood flow to arms)

Aorta
(Main artery off
which other
arteries branch)

Coronary arteries
(blood flow to heart)

Main arteries of
the abdomen
(blood flow to
internal organs)

Femoral arteries
(blood flow to legs)

BLOOD PRESSURES (mmHg)		
	Systolic	Diastolic
At rest:	120 /	80
Vigorous exercise:	160–180 /	75–85

FIGURE 6.9 The main arteries of the cardiovascular system, approximately 100 meters of pressurized tubes. Arterial blood pressure is measured in the right arm at the level of the heart by means of a pressure cuff and gauge.

walls that can reduce their elasticity and narrow the internal diameter of the lumen. Atherosclerosis in a coronary artery can prove lethal, for it threatens the essential supply of oxygen and nutrients to an area of the heart muscle (Figure 6.10). A second condition is excess fat and blood cholesterol. Up to 25 percent of excess body fat is stored within and around the main arteries and the vital organs, where it impedes the normal hemodynamics of the heart and arteries (Figure 6.11). The level of blood cholesterol has been associated with

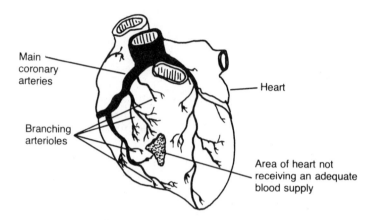

FIGURE 6.10 Effects of partial blockage or complete occlusion in the coronary circulation.

the buildup of these fatty deposits inside arteries. However, cholesterol is a constituent of some important hormones required for normal functioning of the body, and more recent findings[7] suggest that only very high levels of it in the blood constitute a serious risk. A third, very nebulous cause of hypertension is stress, particularly job-related stress.

Millions of North Americans have chosen to regulate high blood pressure with drugs. Many of these persons virtually disregard their diet, live a very sedentary life, yet realize that any sudden activity can injure their heart. Considering their lifestyle, mounting medical costs, and the potential dangers, it seems that healthful exercise augmented by sensible nutrition would prove the better course of action. Properly prescribed activity can help maintain normal blood pressure or help reduce high blood pressure[8]. The exercise stimulus causes vast capillary beds in the active muscles to open up and if the exercise is geared to stressing but never overstressing a particular individual, this repetitive response, combined with a decrease in excess body fat, will help to reduce

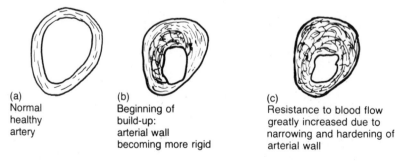

(a)
Normal
healthy
artery

(b)
Beginning of
build-up:
arterial wall
becoming more rigid

(c)
Resistance to blood flow
greatly increased due to
narrowing and hardening of
arterial wall

FIGURE 6.11 Gradual degeneration of an artery as a result of atherosclerosis.

hypertension. Why, then, don't more people choose exercise? Very simply, exercise has always been considered a noxious rather than a positive stimulus. This concept is gradually changing, however, and the positive nature of exercise is one of the main precepts of this text.

Blood. Blood has a number of vital functions throughout the body, one of which, as we have seen, is to distribute oxygen. It accomplishes this with the assistance of a specialized protein called *hemoglobin*, which can combine chemically with oxygen molecules. As with many of the physiological elements of oxygen transport, however, this means of carrying oxygen is potentially hazardous as well as advantageous. That is, blood should be as fluid as possible in order to flow through a vascular system composed of microscopic as well as relatively large tubes. On the other hand, to ensure sufficient oxygen transport for even the mildest activity, there must be approximately 120 to 160 grams of hemoglobin in every liter of our blood. This works out to about 4.6 to 5.4 billion red blood cells per liter of blood—the normal red-blood-cell (RBC) count for women and men, respectively. Blood is therefore quite viscous, which imposes significant hemodynamic limitations upon the heart and vascular system.

By volume, approximately 40 to 45 percent of human blood is protein. This solid portion of the blood, composed primarily of the red blood cells, white blood cells, and platelets, is referred to as the *hematocrit*. The liquid remainder of the blood—the *plasma*—contains dissolved nutrients, minerals, and gases. If the volume of hematocrit in the blood falls much below 40 percent, the result is *anemia*, a condition usually characterized by fatigue and listlessness. On the other hand if it rises much higher than 50 percent—a condition termed *polycythemia*—any potential gain in oxygen-transport capacity will be offset by the additional work required of the heart and vascular system to continually circulate this more viscous blood.

Regular exercise can increase the amount of circulating hemoglobin by as much as 15 grams per liter of blood. This is one of the major causes of the significant improvement in the body's oxygen-transport capacity over the first two months of an exercise prescription. The volume of blood in the vascular system can also increase during this period[9]. Thus, there is no effective increase in hematocrit; in fact, with these two adaptations to regular exercise there is usually a small reduction in the viscosity of the blood.

BODY–TEMPERATURE REGULATION AND EXERCISE

In the muscle cell, many energy transformations are required in order to convert the potential energy in carbohydrates and fats into adenosine triphosphate (ATP). However, not all of the energy is transferred from one stage to the next along the metabolic pathways. But energy is never created or lost, according to the First Law of Thermodynamics; thus energy continually appears in the form of heat (see Figure 5.2) and so is not entirely wasted. The body must maintain its core temperature within an extremely limited range, and as close to 37 degrees centigrade (98.6 degrees Fahrenheit) as possible. The blood circulating through the body can pick up metabolic heat from the areas producing it. This happens in much the same way that coolant circulating through a car's engine absorbs the heat from the block. The circulating blood can then divert the heat to areas of the body that might require it in order to maintain the core temperature. Heat energy not required for temperature maintenance is channeled to the skin's surface, where it can be dissipated into the air. There are several ways in which this dissipation occurs: radiation, convection, conduction, and, our most important mechanism in exercise, evaporation. During evaporation, the sweat glands secrete a thin film of moisture over the surface of the skin; the heat energy is then expended in vaporizing this perspiration.

This basic knowledge of our body's temperature-regulating system is important in exercise prescription because of the interaction of two important factors: (1) the intensity and duration of the activity and (2) the environment in which it is performed. Even in very light activity there can be a three- to fivefold increase in the amount of body heat produced. In heavy, prolonged exercise heat production can increase as much as 15 times. Since exercise is one of the few physiological states in which the body's thermostat will permit the core temperature to rise rather rapidly (Figure 6.12), some of this heat energy can be stored temporarily by the body. The remainder must be dissipated during the exercise. (The heat energy stored during the exercise will eventually have to be dissipated over the one to two hours immediately following the exercise session, as the body's core temperature must return to 37 degrees centigrade.) The temperature and humidity of the environment in which the participant is exercising and into which the heat energy from the exercising muscles must be dissipated dictate the degree to which the thermoregulatory mechanism of the body will be stressed. The two extremes of this environment—heat and humidity at one end and cold water and cold air at the other—must be carefully considered. If they are handled wisely, exercise prescription will prove both safe and comfortable; if disregarded, the consequences can prove uncomfortable, even unsafe (Figure 6.13 and Table 6.2).

1. Exercising in Hot and Humid Environments

The hotter the temperature, the more difficult it becomes for body heat to be released into the atmosphere, and thus the more stress is placed on the body's temperature-regulating mechanisms. The higher the humidity, the more difficult it becomes for the body to vaporize perspiration as well. Therefore, four considerations should temper exercise prescription when exercising in a hot and humid environment (Table 6.2, zone I):

1. One to two hours prior to the exercise session, begin to "waterload" (consume small cups of water every 20 to 30 minutes).

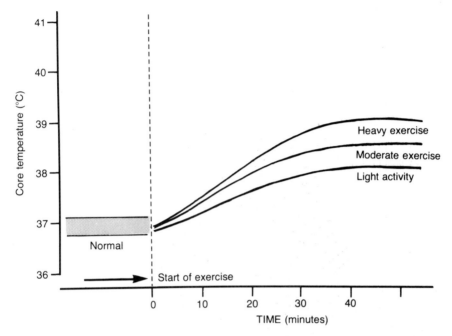

FIGURE 6.12   The rise in the body's core temperature over the initial 20 to 30 minutes of exercise is proportional to the intensity of the activity (light, moderate, or heavy). Normally, core temperature is maintained at 37°C. Some of the heat produced by the working muscles during exercise can be stored temporarily by the body; however, after 20 or 30 minutes *all* of the heat produced must be dissipated, since the body cannot permit the core temperature to rise further.

2. Shorten the warm-up and cool-down as much as possible.
3. Most important, reduce the intensity (e.g., the speed) of the exercise and/ or its duration. In any case it should not exceed half an hour, because of the body-water loss that will have occurred by then.
4. Wear loose-fitting white clothing that exposes much of the shoulders, arms, and legs. The material should be cotton (which assists in the movement of air over the body). In very intense sunlight a sun hat may be worn, for the head is an important heat-dissipating area of the body.

Curiously, over the years sports training has given rise to several mal-practices that should be avoided. During exercise of moderate intensity and at least 10 to 15 minutes duration, sweating is a normal and important part of body-temperature regulation. It is unwise, however, to induce excessive sweating by wearing a rubberized suit or some other body cover, for the body mass lost through sweating is water and *not* fat. Second, if exercise is performed in a hot environment, water intake should *never* be restricted. Third, there is no need to ingest a salt tablet following an exercise session in which the participant has sweated liberally. Because of the additives and preservatives in our foods, our daily diets already contain at least three times the amount of salt we require.

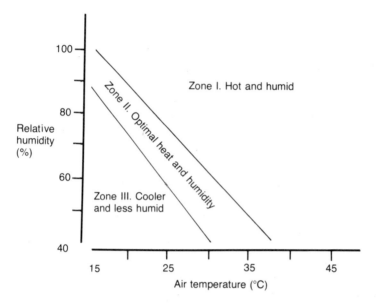

FIGURE 6.13   The three ambient temperature-humidity zones. See Table 6.2.

Finally, if an elevated body temperature or profuse sweating becomes a problem, then the participant is performing too much exercise, and has probably misinterpreted the intent of this text or miscalculated his or her personal prescription (see Part IV).

2. Exercising in Winter and Water Environments

Although the specific cautions related to cold air versus cold water may be different, the principal concern is the same: Is the body heat lost to the environment greater than the heat energy produced by the exercising muscles? Several factors interact to determine the rate of heat loss in cold, but it is important to realize that moderately cold water (≤ 15° centigrade) is potentially more dangerous than even an air temperature close to the freezing point. This is because water is 20 times more efficient than air in dissipating heat from the body's surface. The objective in any cold environment is to normalize the rate of heat lost by the body. One does this by creating a microenvironment around the body with the proper clothing. The following general principles for exercising in cold air (Table 6.2, zone III), should be modified according to the existing *wind-chill factor* (a cold index derived from the air temperature and the wind velocity).

1. Cover and protect as much of the body's surface as prudent, particularly the hands and face as the wind chill dips below zero.

TABLE 6.2 Precautions to Take When Exercising in the Three Heat Zones

Zone	I	II	III
Cautions	waterload before exercising decrease exercise intensity and/or decrease duration to below 30 minutes avoid using nylon material or a rubberized sweat suit	follow normal exercise prescription water ad lib avoid using rubberized sweat suit	cover exposed skin surface: outer covering should be nylon wear wool mittens and wool toque or ski mask avoid using rubberized sweat suit
Clothing	wear white cotton clothing: undershirt, shorts, short sweat socks hat (for shade) is optional	wear cotton T-shirt, shorts, sweat socks sweat shirt or nylon shell optional	under nylon jacket and pants wear: cotton T-shirt under turtleneck sweat shirt (additional sweaters optional) shorts, long sweat socks, long (thermal) underwear, sweat pants optional add these layers of clothing as necessary
Postexercise	do not shower immediately; first permit heart rate and body temperature to decline	normal cool-down routine	get indoors as quickly as possible cool down indoors

2. The outer covering on the arms, legs, and trunk should be lightweight nylon; this will permit sufficient movement of heat from the body into the cold environment but will prevent the wind from chilling the warmed microenvironment inside the clothing.

3. Build up layers of clothing depending upon the severity of the cold. On the trunk and arms, wear a T-shirt, a cotton turtleneck, a sweat shirt if necessary, and sweaters in extreme cold. Cover the lower body with shorts and sweat socks up to the knees, or wear long underwear. Sweat pants can be worn under long-legged nylon outer pants.

4. Be particularly careful in selecting footwear: Will it provide adequate traction in icy conditions, and is it appropriate for slushy days?

Specialized apparel and equipment have been developed for cold-weather sports and activities. Downhill ski suits, cross-country ski apparel, hockey equipment, and so on, have been designed to achieve a balance between the environment and the participant's need to regulate body temperature. The jacket life preserver and the wet suit (the latter for use in very cold water) have been developed for water sports. The wet suit permits a small amount of water to seep inside, where it is quickly warmed by the body, and then insulates this internal layer of water against the external cold of the environment.

NUTRITION: DIET, BODY MASS, AND EXERCISE PRESCRIPTION

Next to oxygen transport, perhaps the most immediate support for the muscles during exercise is provided by nutritional factors. In Chapter 5 we explained the metabolism of carbohydrates and fats in muscles and earlier in this chapter we noted that nutrients are transported by the blood to the muscles. Nutrition involves much more than digestion of the energy substrates, however, and it is surprising, considering the plethora of information available on foods and diets, that most people are uninformed about their own nutrition. Today 50 percent of North Americans are diagnosed by their physicians as overweight—*overfat* would be a more accurate term. At a time when providing food for the world's population has become a problem of the first magnitude, diet clinics all over North America are charging as much as $150 per visit simply to convey some basic information and advice about nutrition. And although our standard of living is the highest in the world, our nutritional affluence is literally killing us. We have the highest mortality rates in the world from heart and vascular diseases, we pay exorbitant morbidity costs, and a significant percentage of our population bears the burden of obesity. To begin this section on the important role that nutrition must play in exercise prescription, we offer eight sample questions that will test your general knowledge of some basic facts of nutrition. To how many of the following questions can you answer 'YES'?

> *Example:* Do you know the first rule for achieving good nutrition?
> YES. (DAILY CONSUMPTION OF A WELL-BALANCED DIET).

YES NO **1.** Can you name the six basic components of a well-balanced diet?

YES NO **2.** Do you know how to estimate your daily caloric (energy) needs?

YES NO **3.** Do you know if your daily calorie intake is made up of 55 percent carbohydrate, 30 percent fat, and 15 percent protein?

YES NO **4.** Do you know if your daily consumption of the water-soluble vitamins is sufficient?

YES NO **5.** Do you know if you eat a nourishing breakfast?

YES NO **6.** Do you know how many calories are stored in one kilogram of fat?

YES NO **7.** Can you accurately estimate the percentage of your body mass that is fat?

YES NO **8.** Do you understand why prescribed exercise, in conjunction with your diet, gives you the best chance for permanently losing and/or controlling your body mass?

(*Note:* "Because exercise uses up calories" is *not* the correct answer!)

If you answered yes to less than 5 of these questions, rate your knowledge of nutrition below average.

The Basics of Nutrition

Nutrition is the general term employed for categorizing the foods we eat and the elements, or nutrients, in food that are essential for health. Nutritional requirements vary greatly with many interacting factors: one's age, gender, size and mass, level of activity, lifestyle, health, and so on. The frequency with which a specific nutrient must be ingested depends upon its rate of utilization and on the body's ability to produce and/or store it. For example, both water and energy substrate are essential for health; however fluids must be constantly consumed, whereas the body can store almost limitless amounts of calories, in the form of fat, as well as obtain energy from alternate sources in the body.

Food requirements have been classified into six essential nutrients: water, carbohydrates, fats, proteins, vitamins, and minerals. The important nutritional facts concerned with each are summarized in Table 6.3.

1. *Water* is the most essential nutrient—in fact it accounts for 60 to 70 percent of our body mass. It is found in all cells and tissues, and there must be a *constant* exchange of water between the body and the environment. Normally we drink the equivalent of 2 to 3 liters of water each day, obtaining it principally from our fluid intake and also from many foods (for example, a stalk of celery is almost 90 percent water). Increased physical activity, particularly in a humid climate, can increase the required volume of fluid intake. On the other hand, dehydrating the body through excessive sweating (in a sauna, by using a rubberized suit, or otherwise) or by water restriction can be dangerous and will achieve only a temporary loss of mass, since the volume of water lost through sweating must be replaced.

2. *Carbohydrates* are obtained from foods of plant origin: vegetables, grains, and fruits. These are the most important foods in our diet, both because of their caloric value and because they provide the majority of our daily requirements of vitamins and minerals. And about 55 percent of our *modest* daily caloric needs should be obtained from these foods. The processing of plant foods, however, can remove many of their nutrients, so it has become common within the food industry to *reenrich* many of their products and then redundantly label the end-product *enriched*. Excessive boiling of vegetables can also remove some of their important nutrients. Carbohydrates obtained from processed products such as refined sugar (table sugar, candy, and so forth) and alcoholic beverages are referred to as *empty calories* because these foods are devoid of additional

TABLE 6.3   General Guidelines for a Well-Balanced Diet

DIETARY COMPONENT	GUIDELINES	DAILY CONSUMPTION
1. WATER	Take in water as required; in a hot environment and/or during exercise increase intake	2–3 liters
		% of energy requirement
2. CARBOHY-DRATES	Increase consumption of complex carbohydrates >40% decrease consumption of empty calories <15%	} 55%
3. FATS	Increase consumption of poly-unsaturated fats >15% Decrease the consumption of satu-rated fats <15%	} 30%
4. PROTEINS	Consume only 1 gram of protein for each kilogram of body weight	(15%*)
5. VITAMINS	Consume water-soluble vitamins (C, B group) daily Only limited storage in body of fat-soluble vitamins (A, D, E) is pos-sible	all of these vitamin and mineral requirements can be obtained only from a *wide variety* of foods
6. MINERALS	24 *essential* minerals, and at least 31 in all, are found in the body	

*Protein requirements are calculated in energy units (calories) but are *not* used as an energy substrate in a well-balanced diet.

nutrients. Therefore, it is a good idea to select complex carbohydrates—those that have nutrient value—and to reduce the consumption of foods that are high only in carbohydrates. For those engaged in an exercise program a *small* daily increase in caloric consumption may be necessary (when a reduction in mass is unnecessary); these calories should be obtained from carbohydrates, not from fats.

3. *Fats* are obtained from animal food sources, principally meat and dairy products, as well as from a limited number of plant food sources. As with the other components of nutrition, there are some basic facts about fats that many people are not aware of. When we consume fats, we are ingesting the richest form of energy. A gram from most fat sources contains more than twice the energy in one gram of carbohydrate. Therefore our daily consumption of fats should be much lower than carbohydrates—only about 30 percent of our total caloric requirement. An important distinction should be made regarding the origin of fats. With few exceptions, animal food sources provide the saturated fats in our diet and plant sources the unsaturated fats. Only the saturated fats increase blood cholesterol, and thus less than half our daily consumption of fats should be saturated fats. The distinction between the fats we consume and the role of our body fat should also be clarified. A modest consumption of fats is essential in our diet; body fat is internally stored energy. Our body has a very finite capacity to store energy in forms other than fat. Therefore the extra calories we consume each day but do not metabolize must be stored as body fat—and we can store a voluminous amount of body fat in a relatively short time. Finally, while fats should provide only 30 percent of our daily caloric needs, most North Americans obtain 40 to 50 percent of their calories from fats. This amount can quickly be reduced if one consumes a minimum of lean meats and more fat-free dairy products.

4. Several classes of *protein* and thousands of complex proteins are found in the body. Protein is present in every cell and tissue, and involved with every regulating process in the body. Obviously it is an essential nutrient, yet it should provide only about 15 percent of our daily caloric requirement. Why? Quite simply, protein is not used as an energy substrate; that is the role of carbohydrates and fats. Thus the confusion for most people regarding their consumption of protein is due to the fact that the daily volume of protein that we require for essential but *nonenergy* purposes is measured in units of *energy* (calories). Another point of confusion for most people is that the sources of protein are almost the same as the sources of fat: animal foods (principally meat, fish, and dairy products), and a limited number of plant foods. Thus the principle that applies to carbohydrate intake (eat foods that provide both carbohydrates *and* minerals and vitamins) has a corollary regarding protein intake: eat foods that contain both fat *and* protein nutrients.

5. *Vitamins* are found in small amounts in almost all of the plant and animal foods we eat. However, improper preparation of foods, particularly the overcooking of vegetables, can greatly reduce their vitamin content. Our need for all vitamins is small but essential, for they play a critical role in the complex biochemical reactions of the body. We require 14 vitamins; for simplification they have been classified as A, the B group, C, D, and E. Unlike carbohydrates, fats, and some proteins, vitamins cannot be synthesized by our body; we must obtain them from external food sources. Thus we must eat a variety of foods to ensure a daily intake of all the vitamins. More important, however, only some of the vitamins can be stored in the body. Vitamins A, D, and E—the *fat-soluble* vitamins—can be stored in very limited quantities in the fat depots of the body; vitamin C and the B group—the *water-soluble* vitamins—cannot, and excess amounts of these vitamins are excreted. Hence a daily intake of the water-soluble vitamins is one of our most important nutritional requirements.

6. Finally, 24 *minerals* that are essential for healthy growth and mainte-nance of the body have been identified; at least 31 are present in the body. Minerals are used by almost every tissue and physiological process in the body. Calcium and phosphorous are the most abundant minerals in the body and are essential for healthy bones and teeth. Calcium is also involved in the mechanism that triggers muscular contraction, as are sodium and potassium, which play an integral role in the conduction of nerve impulses. Iron is the oxygen-carrying element in hemoglobin. Sulphur and magnesium are found in substantial amounts in the body; iodine, zinc, copper, and manganese in much smaller quantities; and molybdenum, selenium, vanadium, chromium, and several other minerals only in traces. Minerals are present in the plant and animal foods we consume —another good reason for consuming a variety of foods.

Personalized Daily Nutrition

By themselves, these basic facts on nutrition have only limited application; now this information must be personalized to enable individuals to modify their own diet. In this section we detail formulas and guidelines for determining personal nutritional requirements in relation to one's age and sex, size and body weight, lifestyle, eating habits, and so on. The first step is to determine daily caloric (energy) expenditure.

Your Daily Energy Expenditure.   You can estimate your average daily caloric expenditure and verify its accuracy by monitoring your body weight over a period of 6 to 8 weeks. If your weight shows only small fluctuations ($\leq$ 1.5 kilograms or 3 pounds) over this period, then your calculations provided an accurate estimate of your caloric expenditure. However, if there was a definite gain or loss of weight by the end of two months, then you should adjust your estimate accordingly (unless, of course, your aim was to lose or gain weight). A number of interacting factors determine your daily caloric expenditure. Chart I includes three major components. The *basal energy component,* which represents the calories required merely to keep your body functioning over a 24-hour period, is influenced by gender and body size. Males require approximately 10 percent more basal energy than females. Larger persons (who have billions of additional body cells) also require greater basal energy. The *lifestyle component* is an estimate of the calories required for carrying out your daily activities. Is your lifestyle *very* sedentary—are you awake 16 to 18 hours per day, asleep 6 to 8 hours, and at work 8 hours at a sedentary job?—or is it more active? The third component of the formula is the *exercise component.* One session of exercise or physical activity, no matter how strenuous it may seem, actually expends relatively few calories—rarely more than 10 or 15 percent of your total energy expenditure for that day. Remember that the calculations in chart I are approximate and are subject to daily variations.

Your Daily Nutritional Intake.   A balanced diet (Figure 6.14) is the basis of good nutrition. It involves two fundamental concepts. First, and of more immediate concern, an energy balance must be maintained. That is, the energy you consume each day must equal your daily energy expenditure. Second, the nutrients your body requires must be consumed on a regular basis. To achieve these nutritional objectives, we classify our foods according to the five basic food groups and then calculate recommended servings (or cups, in the case of liquids). By following the steps outlined below you can determine your daily

CHART I. CALCULATION OF YOUR DAILY CALORIC EXPENDITURE

CALORIES
USED UP
PER 24
HOURS

1. Basal Energy Component

For adult females: multiply 21.7 $\times$ _____
body mass (in kg)

= [ ]

For adult males: multiply 24.1 $\times$ _____
body mass (in kg)

2. Lifestyle Component (calculate only <u>one</u>; each lifestyle assumes 6–8 hours of sleep a day)

A. Sedentary lifestyle (limited standing and walking; no activity)

multiply 0.4 $\times$ _____
(calories calculated in step #1)

B. Active lifestyle (standing, walking, and recreational activities)

multiply 0.5 $\times$ _____
(calories calculated in step #1)

= [ ]

C. Physical labor (employment involving 6 to 8 hours of lifting, loading, shoveling, etc.)

multiply 0.6 $\times$ _____
(calories calculated in step #1)

3. Total Daily Caloric Expenditure: Basal + Lifestyle (add boxes 1 and 2)

= [ ]

4. Exercise Component (assumes the equivalent of 30 minutes of activity or exercise prescription)

multiply 0.12 $\times$ _____
(total from step #3)

= [ ]

5. Total Daily Caloric Expenditure: Basal + Lifestyle + Exercise   = [ ]

DAILY NUTRITIONAL CONSUMPTION:

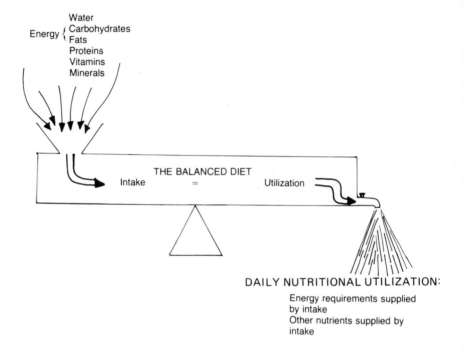

FIGURE 6.14   The concept of a balanced diet. On average, one's daily nutritional intake meets one's daily nutritional requirements.

energy and nutritional requirements. Again, by monitoring your body weight for 6 to 8 weeks, you can make minor modifications in your recommended diet (as described under step 2).

Step 1. Determine Your Balanced Diet

Table 6.4 consists of recommended servings, based upon an individual's caloric requirements, from the five food groups. (If your consumption of empty calories—popularly termed junk foods—is considerable, you should complete step 1A beforehand.) Select the column that corresponds to your total caloric expenditure, as calculated in the preceding section. If that figure falls between two columns, adjust the daily recommended servings from each food group according to step 2. The total number of servings will form the basis for the daily amount of food that you should consume.

Step 1A. Calculate the Empty Calories You Consume

Almost every person consumes empty calories—foods and beverages that supply calories but few essential nutrients. We urge you to minimize their intake or

CHART II. CALCULATION OF EMPTY CALORIES CONSUMED PER DAY

CATEGORY OF FOOD

SUGARS:

    1 tsp. of white sugar   _____

    1 tsp. of jam, syrup   _____

    1 candy (i.e., hard, caramel)   _____

              CATEGORY TOTAL   _____   X 15 Calories   =   [   ]

FATS:

    1 tbsp. cream (½ oz.)   _____

    ½ tbsp. salad dressing, oils   _____

    1 tbsp. gravy, sauce   _____

              CATEGORY TOTAL   _____   X 35 Calories   =   [   ]

BEVERAGES:

  Soft drinks

      1 bottle of pop (10 oz.)   _____

      1 oz. powder mix
      (sweetened)   _____

              TOTAL   _____   X 100 Calories   =   [   ]

  Alcoholic

      1 shot liquor (1½ oz.)   _____

      1 glass wine (4 oz.)   _____

              TOTAL   _____   X 100 Calories   =   [   ]

      1 bottle beer (12 oz.)   _____   X 150 Calories   =   [   ]

SNACKS:

    1 small bag of potato chips   _____

    1 plain chocolate bar   _____

    1 plain doughnut   _____

              CATEGORY TOTAL   _____   X 150 Calories   =   [   ]

DESSERTS:

    1 piece of pie, pastry, cake,
    baked dessert   _____

    6 cookies (@ 50 calories/per)   _____

              CATEGORY TOTAL   _____   X 300 Calories   =   [   ]

              TOTAL EMPTY CALORIES   [   ]
              CONSUMED PER DAY

Table 6.4 Recommended Daily Servings Based on Daily Caloric Expenditure*

FOOD GROUP	IF YOUR DAILY CALORIC EXPENDITURE** IS				
	1000 CALORIES	1500 CALORIES	2000 CALORIES	2500 CALORIES	3000 CALORIES
MEAT	1	1½	2	2½	3
MILK	2	2	3	3	4
VEGETA-BLES	1	2	2	3	4
FRUIT	1	1½	2	2½	3
BREAD and CEREAL	2	3	4	4	5

*Daily recommended servings will provide a well-balanced diet for a healthy adult:
  1 serving from meat group = 2 to 3 ounces lean meat; one egg can be substituted.
  1 serving from milk group = 8 ounces (1 cup).
  1 serving from vegetable group = equivalent of 4 to 8 ounces of raw or cooked vegetables.
  1 serving from fruit group = one average-size piece of fruit (the equivalent of 4 to 8 ounces).
  1 serving from bread and cereal group = 1 slice of bread, 1 roll, etc. (the equivalent of 4 to 8 ounces of grains and cereal foods).
**Adjust your daily caloric expenditure according to the empty calories that you consume each day (step 1A).

Source: Reprinted through the courtesy of the Ministry of Health, Province of Ontario, Canada.

substitute more nutritional foods, yet we realize that these calories are an integral part of the North American diet. Since they are not included in Table 6.4, an adjustment must be made to take into account your daily consumption of empty calories.

Use chart II to calculate your empty calories. For each item estimate the number of servings you consume per day, and enter the numbers in the spaces provided. Total each category, and then multiply by the caloric value per serving. Add up these totals to get your grand total.

Finally, subtract your total of empty calories consumed each day from your daily caloric expenditure, to derive your adjusted value of calories to be supplied by the food groups:

Daily Caloric Expenditure (box 3 or 5 in chart I)

Empty Calories Consumed Per Day (calculated in chart II) —

Calories to be supplied by food groups (adjusted value) =

Use this adjusted value to select the appropriate column in Table 6.4.

Let's work through an example. Assume that your daily energy expenditure is 2500 calories and that in step 1A you calculated that 500 of these calories come from:

2 bottles of beer $\times$ 150 calories = 300 calories

2 bottles of pop $\times$ 100 calories = 200 calories

500 empty calories per day

To achieve caloric balance, you should obtain only 2000 calories per day from the food groups:

$$
\begin{array}{ll}
2500 & \text{calories per day} \\
-500 & \text{empty calories per day} \\
\hline
2000 & \text{calories per day}
\end{array}
$$

Therefore you should use the 2000 calories column in Table 6.4 to determine the number of servings you should consume per day from each food group. That would mean:

meat:	2 servings (approximately 4 to 6 oz. meat)
milk:	3 glasses (24 oz.)
vegetables:	2 normal servings
fruit:	2 normal servings or 2 pieces raw fruit (apple, orange, etc.)
bread and cereal:	4 servings (for example: 1 bowl of cereal, 2 slices of bread, 1 serving of spaghetti or pasta)

Step 2. Adjust Your Recommended Daily Servings

After you have determined your recommended daily servings from each of the food groups, the next step is to suit these dietary requirements to your taste. Are there particular foods you like (such as potatoes every day), or do you prefer a wider variety of foods in your weekly menu? Table 6.5 lists the most common foods we consume from each of the food groups. More important, the foods in each group have been categorized according to their caloric content: lower, medium, or higher. Therefore, if you find, for example, that you are slowly gaining weight, you may still remain on your recommended diet simply by substituting a "medium" for a "higher," or a "lower" for a "medium," food in the same food group.

TABLE 6.5 The Five Food Groups with Relative Caloric Content of Foods

Lower Calorie Foods	Medium Calorie Foods	Higher Calorie Foods
MEAT GROUP		
chicken	beef	meat pies
turkey	lamb	sausage meat
fish	veal	luncheon meats
seafood	pork	nuts; seeds
canned fish	ham	peanut butter
	eggs	chili
	corned beef	bacon
	liver	baked beans
MILK GROUP		
skim milk	whole milk	chocolate milk
two-percent milk	cheese	ice cream
buttermilk	cottage cheese	milk pudding
low-fat cheese	plain yogurt	milk shakes
		cream soups
		instant-breakfast products
		flavored yogurt
VEGETABLE GROUP		
asparagus	beets	lima beans
green and yellow beans	broccoli	corn
bean sprouts	brussels sprouts	potatoes
cabbage	carrots	sweet potato
cauliflower	peas	
celery	pumpkin	
cucumber	spinach	
green pepper	tomatoes and juice	
lettuce	turnip	
mushrooms	winter squash	
radish		
summer squash		
zucchini		
FRUIT GROUP		
watermelon	apples and juice	avocado
	bananas	dried apricot
	berries	dates
	cantaloupe	prunes and juice
	grapefruit and juice	raisins
	oranges and juice	syrup-packed canned fruit
	peaches	
	pears	
	pineapples and juice	
	plums	
BREAD AND CEREAL GROUP		
whole-grain breads	macaroni, spaghetti	pie
enriched breads	egg noodles	cake
whole-grain cereals	pancakes	sweet rolls
unsweetened cereals	waffles	date squares
whole-grain crackers	rice	pastries
plain rolls	sweetened cereals	granola-type cereals
	muffins	
	tea biscuits	
	oatmeal cookies	

Source: Ministry of Health, Province of Ontario, Canada.

Let's consider another example.

Suppose you *slowly* gained weight consuming the recommended diet in the 2000 calories column of the Table 6.4.

Assume also that you do not wish to increase your activity level in order to metabolize this small number of extra calories you consume each day.

Thus a *small* reduction in your caloric consumption is necessary, and you can achieve this without any major alteration in your recommended diet. According to Table 6.5, you could make the following modifications:

Meat Group:
Chicken, turkey, and fish (lower-calorie meats) might be substituted for beef, pork, and ham—still 2 servings per day.

Milk Group:
If you like yogurt, you could substitute plain yogurt for the higher-calorie flavored yogurt.

Vegetable Group:
You could switch to lower-calorie vegetables (asparagus, green and yellow beans, bean sprouts, etc.) and still consume 2 servings per day.

Fruit Group:
There are few lower-calorie foods in this group. However, by reducing calorie intake in the other four groups, you could probably still eat 2 servings of your favorites.

Bread and Cereal Groups:
You could substitute 4 servings per day of whole-grain breads, cereals, plain rolls, etc., for medium- and higher-calorie items.

Body Fat, Body Composition, and Exercise Prescription

Considering the day-to-day variation in both our dietary intake and our activity level, our consumption of nutrients can exceed our physiological needs for them. What happens to nutrients that we consume but do not require or metabolize? Can they adversely affect our health or body composition? Generally, an excess of nonenergy nutrients (vitamins, minerals, and water) are excreted. Unfortunately, the energy-containing nutrients (carbohydrates and fats) cannot be excreted. If there is an excess, it must be stored, and mainly in the form of body fat, since our body can retain only a limited surplus of carbohydrates. And our capacity to store surplus energy in the form of fat is prodigious (see Figure 6.15).

The Role of Body Fat. Essentially our body fat is stored energy, although it serves other physiological functions. A small percentage of body fat (2 to 3 percent), referred to as *essential fat,* is critically important in several physiological functions, including the transmission of nerve impulses, the production of body hormones, and the protection of vital organs. The most accessible site for storage of fat is just below the skin in specialized cells called *adipose tissue.* Fat stored

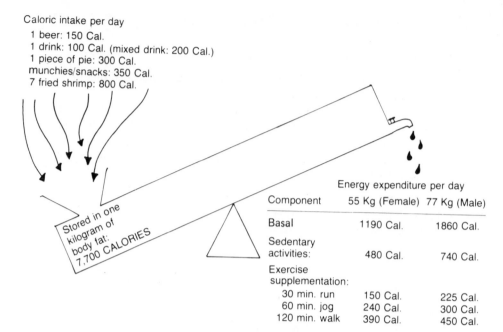

Caloric intake per day
1 beer: 150 Cal.
1 drink: 100 Cal. (mixed drink: 200 Cal.)
1 piece of pie: 300 Cal.
munchies/snacks: 350 Cal.
7 fried shrimp: 800 Cal.

Stored in one kilogram of body fat: 7,700 CALORIES

Energy expenditure per day		
Component	55 Kg (Female)	77 Kg (Male)
Basal	1190 Cal.	1860 Cal.
Sedentary activities:	480 Cal.	740 Cal.
Exercise supplementation:		
30 min. run	150 Cal.	225 Cal.
60 min. jog	240 Cal.	300 Cal.
120 min. walk	390 Cal.	450 Cal.

FIGURE 6.15 The concept of energy imbalance. Daily caloric consumption exceeds daily energy expenditure. The extra calories will be stored as fat.

at these sites is termed *subcutaneous fat*. This method of storage requires three fat molecules to bond chemically; the resulting *triglyceride* molecule can be densely packed into the adipose cell. Fat stored subcutaneously can also serve several important functions:

1. It can give additional shape to the body, for it is outside the muscles and skeleton. In fact, an optimal percentage of body fat, 10 to 15 percent for males and 15 to 22 percent for females, gives the face and various body parts a healthy and attractive appearance.
2. At several locations on the body (such as the buttocks) the subcutaneous fat provides the only cushioning for the underlying muscles and bones.
3. Subcutaneous fat can serve as an insulator, helping the body maintain its core temperature of 37° centigrade in cold weather.

However, these apparent advantages of body fat are non-sequiturs, considering our modern living standards and our sedentary lifestyle. We eat the most nutritious diet in the world. Our society is the most technologically advanced, so just how much energy storage do we need? Every kilogram of body fat contains approximately 7700 calories of stored energy; therefore one kilogram alone could supply our modest energy needs for several days! It is our clothes and homes (centrally heated in winter and air-conditioned in summer) rather than our body fat that primarily protect us against drastic climatic changes. And although optimal subcutaneous fat can enhance the appearance of our body, an abundance of it will progressively misshape the body and place undue stress on the vascular system. Females tend to deposit excess fat disproportionately on their buttocks, breasts, and thighs, and males on their trunk, particularly the abdomen. But each person is unique in this regard, and for this reason spot reduction of fat is one of the cruelest of fitness myths. Exercise (plus diet) will utilize more stored fats from a specific depot in one person, but in a second individual an identical program may mobilize proportionately more stored energy from another locale. Finally, although most excess body fat is stored subcutaneously, up to 25 percent of it is deposited around and within the vital organs, especially the heart and the major arteries. This, combined with our sedentary lifestyle, presents the most life-threatening consequence of excessive body fat for North Americans, for it can initiate a degenerative syndrome that will severely impair vital cardiovascular functions over time.

Analysis of Body Composition. In order to examine body fat, we have subdivided the composition of the body into two basic components: *fat* and *nonfat* (or *lean*). This simple model of body composition permits *quantitative* analysis of body fat. It also isolates two important lean components of the body—the muscles and skeleton. These latter components can only be analyzed *qualitatively*, by anthropometric measurements (our height, body widths, and girths) or through functional analyses (of our flexibility and strength). In order to analyze body composition, a number of criteria have been established for each component. For example, muscular strength is the most trainable physical capacity we possess, and absolute criteria for it have been established according to our sex and age (see Tables 7.6–7.10). Skeletal measurements are determined more by our heredity than by environmental influences. And we use a mix of these two extremes—absolute and subjective criteria—to evaluate other lean body components: the degree of muscle definition, shoulder-to-hip ratio, chest-to-waist ratio. We also use aesthetic criteria. On the other hand, absolute criteria have been established for the fat component of our body: in males 10 to 15 percent of body mass should be fat, in females 15 to 22 percent. Within these ranges individuals should attempt to establish a body mass that they can reasonably expect to maintain over the years. This optimal mass can be easily calculated:

1. Determine lean body mass (nonfat mass):
   Lean body mass (in kg.) =
   $$\left[\text{present body mass (kg.)} - \left(\text{present mass} \times \frac{\% \text{ body fat*}}{100} \right) \right]$$

2. Determine present fat mass:
   $$\text{Fat mass (in kg.)} = \left[\text{total body mass (kg.)} - \text{lean body mass (kg.)} \right]$$

3. Calculate optimal mass:
   a. Optimal fat mass (in kg.) =
   $$\left[\text{lean body mass (kg.)} \times \frac{\text{optimal } \% \text{ body fat**}}{100} \right]$$

* Methods for determining percentage of one's body fat are detailed in Chapter 7.
** For males optimal body fat is 10 to 15 percent; for females 15 to 22 percent.

b. Therefore optimal body mass (in kg.) =

$$\left[\text{lean body mass (in kg.) + optimal fat mass (in kg.)} \right]$$

4. Therefore, the number of kilograms by which the present body mass will have to be reduced =

$$\left[\text{present body mass (kg.)} - \text{calculated optimal mass (kg.)} \right]$$

Exercise Prescription and Body Mass.   Much has been written about exercise as a means of weight control, and much of this writing is confusing. Therefore we attempt here to present a clear and concise model for either losing body mass or controlling it. The most important point to remember is that even a substantial amount of exercise accounts for only 10 to 15 percent of your daily caloric expenditure (see Figure 6.15, lower right-hand corner). Therefore controlling your intake of carbohydrates and fats is mandatory. Furthermore, even under strict dietary restraints it requires time—weeks, not days—to expend the calories stored in 1 kilogram of body fat. For example, if your daily energy expenditure was 2567 calories, it would require three days of fasting to utilize the 7700 calories stored in one kilogram of fat. But such an approach is impossible because people must eat daily in order to obtain essential vitamins and minerals. Thus, the most controlled diet, even with the aid of exercise, can metabolize stored energy only at a limited rate.

a. Establishing a Negative Energy Balance.   In this text we are proposing a change in lifestyle, and this implies *long-range* objectives and planning. This approach is particularly applicable to losing, then finally controlling, one's body mass. At birth and through their adolescence years, people weigh many kilograms less than their adult weight. It took time to accumulate the 7700 calories stored in each kilogram of excess body fat, and it will take time to lose them. Thus a long-range approach is mandatory. The first step is to determine the total amount of body mass that you must lose. You should plan to reduce at a rate *no faster than 0.5 kilograms* (about 1 pound) *per week.* If you lose more than this, your limited food intake may eventually cause deficiencies in some of the essential nutrients. This rate corresponds to a MAXIMUM *negative energy balance* of −550 calories per day. Therefore, the number of weeks over which you must remain in negative energy balance can be calculated, and by regularly monitoring your body mass you can check on your progress. The following example illustrates this calculation.

Subject: male, age 25
  body mass = 100 kg. (222 lbs.)
  percent body fat = 25% (as determined by evaluation in Chapter 7)

1. Objective: to reduce body fat to optimal; 12% has been selected as optimal.

2. Calculation of optimal body mass (see preceding section):

$$\text{lean body mass} = \left[100 \text{ kg.} - \left(100 \text{ kg.} \times \frac{25\% \text{ fat}}{100} \right) \right] = 75 \text{ kg.}$$

Thus at 12% body fat,

$$\text{optimal fat mass} = \left[75 \text{ kg.} \times \left(\frac{12\% \text{ fat}}{100}\right)\right] = 9 \text{ kg.}$$

Therefore, optimal body mass = 84 kg.

3. Reduction in present body mass required:
(100 kg. − 84 kg.) = 16 kg.

4. Long-range diet plan: to lose 0.25 kg. per week; thus the duration of the plan will be
[16 kg. ÷ 0.25] = 64 weeks (1 year and 3 months)

5. Establishment of a negative energy balance (for diet only):
If 7700 calories are stored in 1 kg. of body fat,
then 7700 × 0.25 kg. per week = 1925 calories per week
1925 calories per week ÷ 7 days = 275 calories per day

Therefore, by utilizing Table 6.4, this individual can establish a diet in which he will expend 275 calories per day more than he will consume.

In summary: This person can now make a schedule for the next year and three months, calculating what his body weight should be throughout this period, based on a weight loss of one kilogram every four weeks. By monitoring his mass he can determine if his diet requires minor (or even major) adjustments according to Table 6.5.

b. The Role of Exercise Prescription in Controlling Body Mass. When one is attempting to lose or control body mass, the main purpose of prescribed exercise is not the expenditure of a large number of calories, since each session of an exercise prescription is not intended to utilize a large amount of energy. But over an extended period, one year for instance, an exercise prescription will expend thousands of additional calories. During the initial 2 or 3 weeks of a crash diet, on the other hand, the reduction in body mass can occur surprisingly fast. However, this can prove deceiving, since a substantial volume of body water is being lost from the lean body tissues, particularly the large muscles. When the diet is terminated this water loss is replenished, and this can prove discouraging. Prescribed exercise combined with sensible dieting can minimize this effect. Moreover, exercise performed two hours before eating suppresses the sensation of hunger.

How effective can an exercise prescription be in losing or controlling body mass? If our subject in the previous example elected to commence a personalized exercise prescription (see Chapter 8) in order to lose 275 calories a day, he would have the following options:

1. More active lifestyle; no change in his time schedule. No change in his normal diet would be required. Instead, a 30-minute exercise prescription would expend the 275 calories. Or an alternate activity (see Chapter 9) could be prescribed (for example, 1 hour of walking per day) that would expend the 275 calories. This prescription would have to be carried out over 64 weeks.

2. A combination of more active lifestyle and modification of diet; no change in time schedule. The person need only reduce his food intake minimally, by 100 calories per day, and then through exercise prescription expend only 175 calories per day (a 35-minute walks, 20 minutes of exercise, or an equivalent

alternative activity). Again, the program would have to be carried out over 64 weeks.

3. A combination of more active lifestyle and modification of diet; reduction in schedule. If the subject combines a moderate 275 calorie-per-day reduction in dietary intake and begins an exercise prescription that will utilize 275 calories per day, then his schedule for losing the required 16 kilograms can be reduced from 64 weeks to 32 weeks. This rate of weight loss—550 calories per day, or 3850 calories per week—would be the recommended maximum, and if carefully monitored would reduce body fat (and mass) at a rate of 0.5 kilogram per week.

ADDITIONAL CONSIDERATIONS RELATED TO EXERCISE PRESCRIPTION

There are several factors that influence our muscular activity but are involved less directly in it than the three physiological functions already discussed in this chapter. The importance of these additional factors in exercise prescription can be gauged by the degree to which each affects our physical vigor, our exercise capacities, or our general health. The majority of texts on fitness fail to emphasize that these factors can be divided into two categories: those over which we have little control, such as our sex, hereditary traits, and age, and those we can influence significantly, especially our lifestyle.

Effects of Sex, Heredity, and Age

These three factors exert a major influence on our physical potentials. Even so, they have little bearing on the sedentary but healthy adult's ability to improve his or her exercise capacity. Although there are basic differences between the exercise capacities of males and females, both will react positively to exercise prescription and experience comparable physiological improvements[10]. And although a young adult's exercise potential is greater than an older person's, people well into their 60s can experience significant physiological improvements from prescribed exercise, according to recent research[11].

Sex. On average, the body composition of the adult female is slightly shorter (by 11 centimeters) and lighter (by 15 kilograms) than that of the male. More significant are the gender differences in disposition of lean and fat. The lean body mass of females is about 20 kilograms less than that of males, primarily because of their smaller muscles. On a strength-per-kilogram basis, however, females are the equal of males, and they will experience the same percentage of improvement in their strength from a correctly prescribed exercise program. On the other hand, females possess 3 to 7 kilograms more body fat than males. However, it would be inadvisable, from the standpoint of both health and aesthetics, for females to reduce their fat component disproportionately, because specific hormones (such as estrogen) that control the menstrual cycle must be synthesized in the adipose tissue. Recently, amenorrhea has become a concern among elite female performers who must maintain a minimum of body fat, such as gymnasts, track athletes, and ballet dancers[12]. However, gynecological problems need not arise in the course of prescribed exercise, which can be performed safely during all phases of the menstrual cycle. In addition, the more physically fit female is apt to experience fewer problems during pregnancy and parturition. The most significant difference between adult males and females that will influence their exercise prescription is their maximal capacity for transporting oxygen (see Figure 6.16). On average, that of females is 10 percent lower. Since aerobic exercise is prescribed partly on the basis of maximal oxygen capacity (see Chapter 8), the intensity and duration of exercise prescribed for females can be reduced up to 10 percent.

Heredity. Humans are born with a multitude of inherited characteristics. Eye and hair color, height, and facial features are obvious hereditary traits, but the influence of heredity on disposition, sense of humor, and intelligence is much more obscure. Most people are totally unaware of their physiological endowment, and even when they learn that a close relative has a heart problem or vascular disease the hereditary implications are generally not appreciated. Stated simply, we inherit specific physiological potentials. The handful of great endurance runners were fortunate enough to inherit a vastly superior oxygen-transport system. The majority of people are born with a healthy system; and unfortunately some people inherit a system with potential defects. On the other hand, exercise prescription can be a great help in maximizing one's hereditary potential (see Figure 6.17), and that is the best anyone can hope to achieve. In healthy but

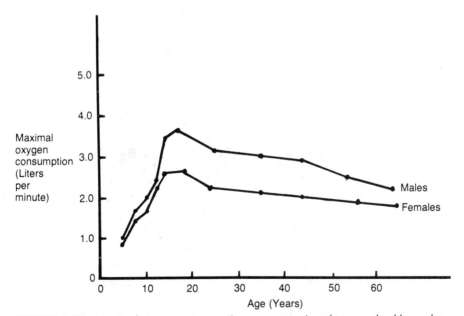

FIGURE 6.16 Maximal oxygen consumption—a comparison between healthy males and females, ages 4–65. *Source*: Adapted from P.-O. Astrand and K. Rodahl, *Textbook of Work Physiology*. Copyright 1970 by McGraw-Hill Inc. and used with the permission of McGraw-Hill Inc.

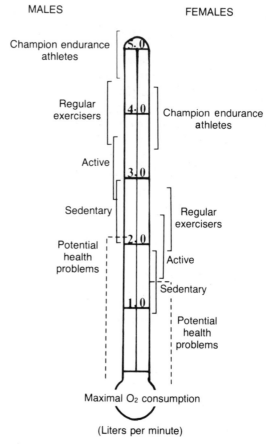

MALES

FEMALES

Champion endurance
athletes

Regular
exercisers

Champion endurance
athletes

Active

Sedentary

Regular
exercisers

Potential
health
problems

Active

Sedentary

Potential
health
problems

Maximal O₂ consumption

(Liters per minute)

FIGURE 6.17 Interactive effects of heredity and exercise prescription. The capacity of one's oxygen-transport system, as measured by maximal oxygen consumption, can be improved by as much as 15 percent; however, one's heredity potential imposes absolute limits on improvement.

sedentary adults, maximal oxygen consumption can be improved up to 15 percent with prescribed exercise. Persons with superior maximal oxygen capacity will need more time and effort to attain an improvement of 15 percent, whereas the obese or the very unfit can expect an improvement of up to 25 percent when they embark upon an exercise program.

Age. Far too many persons accept aging as something over which they can exert little control, mentally or physically. Not only are the authors of this text categorically opposed to this way of thinking, most readers will discover they are as well. Our lives are a conglomeration of mental and emotional characteristics, social and cultural experiences, our physical and physiological makeup, our values and beliefs, and several other major human characteristics. These various facets cannot possibly age at identical rates. For example, many adults "think young," or at least do not adhere to the standards and beliefs that characterize their chronological contemporaries. Aging is regarded primarily as a physical phenomenon, yet we are all aware of persons in their 20s who appear more like 40, as well as 60-year-olds who act, feel, and look 40. This is usually credited to one's mental outlook or explained by clichés (you're only as old as you feel).

However, the explanation does have a physical basis, one that has been repeatedly shown experimentally. Figure 6.16 documents the decline in exercise capacity for males and females in terms of maximal oxygen consumption. We can see that the average male and female of age 40 can consume 3.1 and 2.2 liters of oxygen per minute, respectively. Independent of age and gender, the limit of improvement of maximal oxygen consumption is about 15 percent, and with prescribed exercise this improvement is attainable. Thus, if the average 40-year-old male and female were to attain this improvement, their maximal oxygen capacities would increase to 3.6 and 2.5 liters per minute, values characteristic of men and women in their early 20s. Therefore an exercise prescription accompanied by improvements in flexibility, musculature, and body composition can *at the very least* retard the physiological effects of aging. Conversely, if average 40 year-olds assumed a very sedentary lifestyle and their maximal oxygen consumption *declined* 15 percent (to 2.6 liters O_2 per minute for males and 1.9 for females), then in a relatively short period their physiological functioning would be similar to that of men and women 55 to 60 years of age.

Lifestyle Factors

Among the areas of our life over which we wield some control—and there are many of them—several can directly influence our health and physical vigor. Perhaps the most important of these are the habits and routine that we broadly categorize as our lifestyle.

Inactivity vs. Overactivity. The negative connotations associated with "exercise" may be attributed, first, to individuals who want to become fit in a week or two regardless of discomfort or fatigue and, second, to fitness experts who permit, even encourage, this approach. The objective of exercise prescription is to bring physical activity back into one's lifestyle, and each individual must opt for a personal choice. Physical activity used to be fun—it can be again! For the sedentary person to make such a lifestyle decision—and it is a gradual commitment for most—the successive phases of the exercise prescription must prove intrinsically rewarding. And what is the hurry in any case, particularly if the prescription proves to be a lifelong commitment?

There are three main causes of overactivity among individuals embarking upon a fitness program. First, whether from poor counseling or out of eagerness, many persons begin too quickly. This is absolutely not necessary; follow the model developed in this text. Second, some people attain a certain level of fitness and then conclude that if a little is good, more should prove better. In the case of physical exercise, this will lead over time to generalized fatigue. Finally, there are the cultists who are constantly driving to improve their fitness. But this is impossible once they have achieved their potential level, because each person has a hereditary limitation to his or her level of fitness. The result of such fanaticism is discomfort, and perhaps injury if chronic pain is ignored. Ironically, their lives will also suffer in other aspects, whereas the reason they originally embarked on a fitness program was to improve the quality of their lifestyle.

The symptoms of overactivity are generalized fatigue lasting long after the end of the exercise session and perhaps localized pain in muscles or joints. There is an immediate remedy: reduce the intensity, the duration, or the number of sessions per week of your prescription. Reducing exercise intensity achieves the best result. Limiting the distance run or the length of the session can also prove effective. Nor should one hesitate to reduce the frequency of exercise. If, for example, 5 formal exercise sessions are spread over 2 weeks, this allows 3-day periods to be interspersed between several of the sessions. (This is further detailed in the section on aerobic exercise in Chapter 8.)

Stress vs. Relaxation.   Exercise and stress have a reciprocal relationship. Stress can affect both our lifestyle and exercise capacity, and a positive role for exercise in stress management has recently been documented. *Stress* is any external stimulus that precipitates internal physical, neural, and biochemical reactions. Almost every event in one's life can be included under this working definition. However, as Dr. Selye emphasized through his pioneering research three decades ago, there are positive and negative stresses. It has always been believed that activity provided a positive stress, but this had never been substantiated scientifically. Today we know that many hormones are released into our body in response to any event or situation that we interpret as stressful. And while the results are still inconclusive, recent research has revealed two positive adaptations of our body to the stress of exercise. First, when we exercise, opiatelike chemicals called *endorphins* are released into our blood and brain[13]. Second, persons who exercise regularly tend to have higher endorphin levels in their blood following exercise[14,15]. Endorphins relax the body and promote a sensation of euphoria. Potentially, then, exercise can help us relax, even though physical activity is interpreted by the body as a stress. A primary objective of an exercise prescription is to exert a positive stress—never an excessive stress—by keeping the exercise stimulus well within the capacities of the participant. We cannot avoid stress, particularly in North American society, and in fact we require this stimulation for normal growth and health, just as we need relaxation, rest, and sleep. Achieving a balance between these extremes, consciously or unconsciously, is the goal toward which each individual strives. And although the experimental evidence is still incomplete, it appears that correctly prescribed exercise can help us achieve such a balance.

Tobacco and Alcohol.   No commentary on exercise prescription and fitness would be complete without re-emphasis of the negative consequences of tobacco and alcohol use. Apart from reasons of social conformity or personal gratification, there is little to justify the habitual use of these chemicals. The potential health hazards resulting from long-term use have been well documented. However, information on their short-term effects is less appreciated; in fact the short-term effects of both tobacco and alcohol seem almost negligible—certainly fleeting. Even the governments of the United States and Canada sanction widespread advertising by the manufacturers of these products, though advertising of tobacco products through specific media is now restricted.

Why would anyone intentionally inhale tobacco smoke into his or her lungs when thousands of persons are stricken with lung disease every year through no fault of their own, and when millions of people must endure the air pollution in our major cities. The lungs' small air passages involuntary constrict when exposed to the irritants in smoke. As a result, the smoker will experience difficulty in breathing even during mild exertion. Inhaling cigarette smoke places harsh chemicals such as nicotinic acid near one of the most delicate tissues in our body—the walls of the alveoli, through which gas exchange must occur. The carbon monoxide in tobacco smoke saturates the hemoglobin in our blood, impairing its vital role in oxygen transport. Smoking artificially elevates the heart rate by 10 to 20 beats per minute, and reduces maximal exercise capacity. The most recent reports on smoking emphasize that filter cigarettes do little to alleviate this chain of events[16]. In the short or long term, prescribed exercise is incompatible with tobacco smoking: exercise prescription places a healthful stress upon the physiological systems of the body, whereas the effects of tobacco smoke are diametrically opposed; exercise can be an important aid to improved health, but the constituents of smoke cannot possibly provide any health benefits.

For the nonaddicted, consumption of alcohol is a social phenomenon rather than a nutritional necessity. The food value in any alcoholic drink is limited to its fluid intake and its high caloric content, mainly carbohydrates, since all forms of alcohol lack protein, vitamins, and minerals. Thus, excessive intake of alcohol can cause an imbalance in our daily nutrition. First, the excessive fluid intake combined with the diuretic effects of alcohol can lead to dehydration and the excretion of specific electrolytes, which in turn precipitate a mineral imbalance. Second, since our daily requirement of the various nutrients remains unchanged, we must consume additional food in order to meet our nutritional necessities. Finally, alcohol is a depressant that, unfortunately, acts upon the centers of inhibition of the brain. The result is something like removing the brake pedal from an automobile while leaving the accelerator intact. Judgment, motor function, and spatial awareness are progressively impaired. Only a very moderate level of alcoholic consumption (less than 200 calories per day) is compatible with exercise prescription, when:

1. only 15 percent of one's daily caloric expenditure is utilized in exercise;
2. water balance is vitally important to body-temperature regulation during exercise;
3. the activity requires judgment and coordination, and a clear head on the part of the participant if he or she is to appreciate its exhilarating effect.

REFERENCES

1. Alf Holmgren and Per-Olof Astrand, "D_L and the Dimensions and Functional Capacities of the O_2 Transport System in Humans," *Journal of Applied Physiology,* 21, (1966), 1463–70.

2. C. T. M. Davies and A. V. Knibbs, "The Effects of Intensity, Duration and Frequency of Effort on Maximum Aerobic Power Output," *Internationale Zeitschrift für Angewandte Physiologie,* 26 (1968), 272–78.

3. J. M. Thomson, J. A. Dempsey, L. W. Chosy, W. T. Shahidi, and W. G. Reddan, "Oxygen Transport and Oxyhemoglobin Dissociation During Prolonged Muscular Work," *Journal of Applied Physiology,* 37 (1974), 658–64.

4. Jere H. Mitchell, Brian J. Sproule, and Carleton B. Chapman, "The Physiological Meaning of the Maximal Oxygen Intake Test," *Journal of Clinical Investigation,* 37 (1958), 538–47.

5. Bruce J. Martin, Kenneth E. Sparks, Clifford W. Zwillich, and John V. Weil, "Low Exercise Ventilation in Endurance Athletes," *Medicine and Science in Sports,* 11 (1979), 181–85.

6. Michael L. Pollock, "The Quantification of Endurance Training Programs," *Exercise and Sports Sciences Review,* 1 (1973), 155–88.

7. P. J. Jenkins, R. W. Harper, and P. J. Nestel, "Severity of Coronary Atherosclerosis Related to Lipoprotein Concentration," *British Medical Journal,* 2 (1978), 388–91.

8. James Scheuer and Charles M. Tipton, "Cardiovascular Adaptations to Training," *Annual Review of Physiology,* 39 (1977), 221–51.

9. Bengt Saltin, "Physiological Effects of Physical Conditioning," *Medicine and Science in Sports,* 1 (1969), 50–56.

10. L. H. Getchell and J. C. Moore, "Physical Training: Comparative Responses of Middle-Aged Adults," *Archives of Physical Medicine and Rehabilitation,* 56 (1975), 250–54.

11. M. L. Pollock, et al., "Physiologic Responses of Men 49 to 65 years of Age to Endurance Training," *Journal of the American Geriatrics Society,* 24 (1976), 97–104.

12. Rose E. Frisch, et al., "Delayed Menarche and Amenorrhea of College Athletes in Relation to Age of Onset of Training," *Journal of the American Medical Association,* 246 (1981), 1559–63.

13. David Pargman and Michele C. Baker, "Running High: Enkephalin Indicated," *Journal of Drug Issues,* 10 (1980), 341–49.

14. Danial B. Carr, et al., "Physical Conditioning Facilitates the Exercise-Induced Secretion of Beta-Endorphin and Beta-Lipotropin in Women," *New England Journal of Medicine,* 305 (1981), 560–63.

15. Peter A. Farrell, et al., "Increases in plasma β-endorphin/β-lipotropin immunoreactivity after treadmill running in humans." *Journal of Applied Physiology: Respiratory, Environmental and Exercise Physiology,* 52 (1982), 1245–49.

16. David W. Kaufman, Susan P. Helmrich, Lynn Rosenberg, Olli S. Miettinen, and Samuel Shapiro, "Nicotine and Carbon Monoxide Content of Cigarette Smoke and the Risk of Myocardial Infarction in Young Men," *New England Journal of Medicine,* 308 (1983), 409–13.

7

Personal Fitness Evaluation

INTRODUCTION

Those persons who are physically active and show no signs of contraindications to exercise can safely use a reasonable exercise program to increase their habitual levels of physical activity [1]. Physically inactive individuals and persons over 30 should have a thorough medical examination before assessing their fitness and beginning an exercise program.

We begin this chapter with a questionnaire that will evaluate your readiness for physical activity. You should complete it before proceeding with the fitness evaluation. We then describe techniques for assessing five important parameters of physical fitness:*

A. anthropometry and body composition
B. posture
C. flexibility
D. muscular endurance and strength
E. aerobic capacity

* The techniques for assessing these parameters are adapted from *Standardized Test of Fitness: Operations Manual.* Courtesy Fitness and Amateur Sport Canada.

Individual Personal Profiles are determined for each fitness parameter, then your overall physical fitness is evaluated from these individual Profiles.

PAR-Q EVALUATION

The Physical Activity Readiness Questionnaire[2] is designed to help you help yourself. Many health benefits are associated with regular exercise, and the completion of PAR-Q is a sensible first step to take if you are planning to increase the amount of physical activity in your life. For most people physical activity should not pose any problem or hazard. PAR-Q has been designed to identify the small number of adults for whom physical activity might be inappropriate or who should have medical advice concerning the type of activity most suitable for them. Common sense is your best guide in answering these few questions. Read them carefully and answer them as they apply to you.

YES NO **1.** Has your doctor ever said you have heart trouble?

YES NO **2.** Do you frequently have pains in your heart and chest?

YES NO **3.** Do you often feel faint or have spells of severe dizziness?

YES ₁ NO **4.** Has a doctor ever said your blood pressure was too high?

YES NO **5.** Has your doctor ever told you that you have a bone or joint problem such as arthritis that has been aggravated by exercise, or might be made worse with exercise?

YES NO **6.** Is there a good physical reason not mentioned here why you should not follow an activity program even if you wanted to?

YES NO **7.** Are you over age 65 and not accustomed to vigorous exercise?

If you have answered yes to one or more quesions, and if you have not seen your personal physician recently, you should consult with him or her *before* completing the fitness evaluation in this chapter and/or increasing your physical activity. Explain to your doctor the question(s) to which you answered yes in the PAR-Q. After obtaining a medical evaluation, ask your Physician about your suitability for either:

1. unrestricted physical activity, probably on a gradually increasing basis; or
2. restricted or supervised activity that will meet your specific needs, at least to begin with, if appropriate programs or special services are available in your community.

On the other hand, if you were able to answer no to all the questions, you can be reasonably sure of your present suitability to, first, complete the personal fitness evaluation which follows, and then, based on the results, to develop your *personalized* fitness prescription in Chapter 8. Finally, if you have a temporary minor illness, such as a common cold, it would probably be preferable to postpone the fitness evaluation until you feel better.

A. ANTHROPOMETRIC EVALUATION AND BODY–FAT PROFILE

Two areas of body composition are particularly appropriate for fitness analysis prior to the prescription of exercise. First, the basic *anthropometric measurements* of the body should be recorded: standing height, body mass, and girth measurements (arm, chest, abdominal, gluteal, and thigh circumferences). Throughout the exercise program you can quickly retake these measurements in order to periodically evaluate your progress. Second, the *percentage of body fat* should be determined, and then periodically recalculated after the exercise prescription has been put into practice. One of the best methods for determining this percentage is the caliper method. A skinfold caliper is used to quickly and accurately measure skinfold thickness at four sites on the right side of the body: the biceps and triceps on the right arm and the subscapular and supra-iliac skinfolds. You can then use these measurements to calculate the percentage of your body fat, according to Tables 7.1 and 7.2. An alternate method for determining body fat

TABLE 7.1   Conversion of Total Skinfold Measurements to Percentage of Body Fat

Total Skinfolds (mm)	Percentage of Body Fat							
	Males (age)				Females (age)			
	17–29	30–39	40–49	50+	16–29	30–39	40–49	50+
15	4.8	—	—	—	10.5	—	—	—
20	8.1	12.2	12.2	12.6	14.1	17.0	19.8	21.4
25	10.5	14.2	15.0	15.6	16.8	19.4	22.0	24.0
30	12.9	16.2	17.7	18.6	19.5	21.8	24.5	26.6
35	14.7	17.7	19.6	20.8	21.5	23.7	26.4	28.5
40	16.4	19.2	21.4	22.9	23.4	25.5	28.2	30.3
45	17.7	20.4	23.0	24.7	25.0	26.9	29.6	31.9
50	19.0	21.5	24.6	26.5	26.5	28.2	31.0	33.4
55	20.1	22.5	25.9	27.9	27.8	29.4	32.1	34.6
60	21.2	23.5	27.1	29.2	29.1	30.6	33.2	35.7
65	22.2	24.3	28.2	30.4	30.2	31.6	34.1	36.7
70	23.1	25.1	29.3	31.6	31.2	32.5	35.0	37.7
75	24.0	25.9	30.3	32.7	32.2	33.4	35.9	38.7
80	24.8	26.6	31.2	33.8	33.1	34.3	36.7	39.6
85	25.5	27.2	32.1	34.8	34.0	35.1	37.5	40.4
90	26.2	27.8	33.0	35.8	34.8	35.8	38.3	41.2
95	26.9	28.4	33.7	38.6	35.6	36.5	39.0	41.9
100	27.6	29.0	34.4	37.4	36.4	37.2	39.7	42.6
105	28.2	29.6	35.1	38.2	37.1	37.9	40.4	43.3
110	28.8	30.1	35.8	39.0	37.8	38.6	41.0	43.9
115	29.4	30.6	36.4	39.7	38.4	39.1	41.5	44.5
120	30.0	31.1	37.0	40.4	39.0	39.6	42.0	45.1
125	30.5	31.5	37.6	41.1	39.6	40.1	42.5	45.7
130	31.0	31.9	38.2	41.8	40.2	40.6	43.0	46.2
135	31.5	32.3	38.7	42.4	40.8	41.1	43.5	46.7
140	32.0	32.7	39.2	43.0	41.3	41.6	44.0	47.2

TABLE 7.2 Percentile Scores for Body-Fat Percentage

Males (age)					PERCENTILE SCORE	Females (age)				
17–19	20–29	30–39	40–49	50+		17–19	20–29	30–39	40–49	50+
7.6	9.9	10.5	11.0	13.7	100	9.8	10.0	9.2	10.2	11.6
8.8	11.1	15.2	16.9	19.2	95	15.1	15.3	15.0	16.1	17.2
10.3	12.6	16.1	18.1	20.3	90	16.2	16.3	16.1	17.2	18.4
11.2	13.5	17.3	19.5	21.7	85	17.5	17.6	17.6	18.7	19.9
12.0	14.2	18.0	20.4	22.5	80	18.3	18.3	18.4	19.5	20.8
12.7	14.9	18.6	21.2	23.2	75	18.9	19.0	19.1	20.3	21.6
13.3	15.4	19.2	21.8	23.8	70	19.5	19.5	19.8	20.9	22.3
13.9	16.1	19.6	22.4	24.3	65	20.0	20.0	20.4	21.5	22.8
14.5	16.6	20.1	23.0	24.9	60	20.6	20.6	21.0	22.1	23.5
15.1	17.2	20.5	23.5	25.4	55	21.1	21.0	21.5	22.6	24.0
15.7	17.7	21.0	24.1	25.9	50	21.6	21.5	22.0	23.2	24.6
16.2	18.3	21.5	24.7	26.4	45	22.1	22.0	22.6	23.7	25.2
16.9	18.9	21.9	25.2	26.9	40	22.5	22.5	23.1	24.3	25.8
17.5	19.5	22.4	25.8	27.5	35	23.1	23.0	23.7	24.9	26.4
18.2	20.1	22.8	26.3	28.0	30	23.6	23.5	24.3	25.4	27.0
18.9	20.9	23.4	27.0	28.7	25	24.2	24.1	24.9	26.1	27.7
19.8	21.8	24.0	27.8	29.3	20	24.9	24.7	25.6	26.8	28.4
21.4	23.3	24.7	28.6	30.2	15	25.6	25.5	26.5	27.7	29.3
22.6	24.4	25.9	30.1	31.6	10	27.0	26.8	27.9	29.1	30.9
23.2	25.9	26.8	31.2	32.6	5	28.0	27.8	29.1	30.3	32.1
27.1	32.9	34.2	37.2	38.2	0	33.3	32.9	34.9	36.2	38.2

is described in case calipers are not available. Record all data from this section in score sheet A, page 119.

1. Anthropometric Measurements

Anthropometric dimensions provide information on the general external morphology of the body as well as an indirect means for assessing internal body composition. Although they appear relatively simple, the majority of these determinations must be carefully recorded, since there are variations between repeated measurements.

Procedure for recorder:
1. Sequentially record mass, length, girth, and width measurements.
2. Make duplicate measurements and average them. However, if the second measure is not within 5 percent of the first, record a third measurement and then average the two closest measures.
3. Enter final measurements in score sheet A.

Equipment and Personnel:
sliding meter-stick caliper
flexible (plastic or linen) tape measure
weight scale
apparel: shorts for males
        shorts and halter top or two-piece suit for females
a person to take and record the measurements

Standing Height. Position the tape against a wall. Ensure that the tape is perfectly straight and even with the floor (Figure 7.1). Measure to the highest point on the top of the head, and measure to the nearest 0.2 centimeter. The subject must be barefoot and have the back square against the wall tape, the

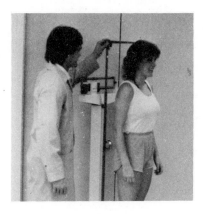

FIGURE 7.1
Standing height.

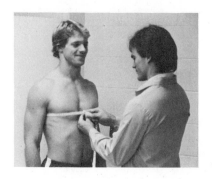

FIGURE 7.2
Chest circumference—male.

heels together, the body stretched upward to the fullest extent, the shoulders relaxed, and the arms stretched downward.

Body Mass.   Ensure that the scale is on a hard, flat surface. Measure body mass to the nearest 0.5 kilogram.

Body Girths.   Ensure that the tape is located in accordance with Figures 7.2–7.6 and the following instructions. Attempt to use the same tension on the tape for all measurements. Measure to the nearest 0.5 centimeter.

Left- and Right-Arm Circumferences.   Arms must hang relaxed at the sides. Measure the circumference of the upper arms at the midpoint of the biceps.

Chest Circumference (Males).   Measure the unclothed chest, at the level of the nipples, at the end of normal expiration (Figure 7.2).

Chest Circumference (Females).   Measure the chest, clothed in a halter top or swimsuit, at the end of normal expiration (Figure 7.3).

Abdominal Circumference.   Measure the unclothed abdomen at the level of the umbilicus (Figure 7.4).

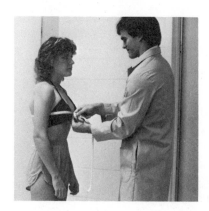

FIGURE 7.3
Chest circumference—female.

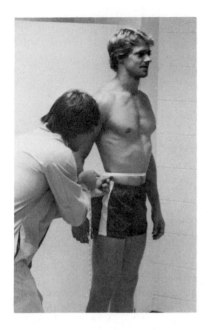

FIGURE 7.4
Abdominal circumference.

Gluteal (Buttock) Circumference. With the subject standing, measure from the side at the normal protrusion of the gluteals and anteriorly at the level of the symphysis pubis (Figure 7.5).

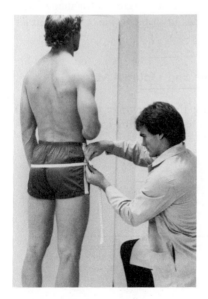

FIGURE 7.5
Gluteal circumference.

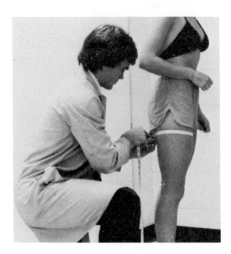

FIGURE 7.6
Thigh circumference.

Left- and Right-Thigh Circumferences. With the subject standing, measure the unclothed thigh just below the gluteal furrow at the maximal girth (Figure 7.6).

Body Widths. Using the sliding meter-stick caliper (Figure 7.7), measure to the nearest 0.5 centimeter.

Shoulder Width. Measure the distance between the lateral aspects of the acromial processes (Figure 7.8).

Hip Width. Measure the distance between the lateral margins of the iliac crests. You may have to apply pressure with the caliper in order to make firm contact with the bones (Figure 7.9).

2. Calculation of Body-Fat Percentage and Optimal Mass

We present two methods for calculating the percentage of body fat: (a) from the total of the four skinfold measurements, and (b) from selected anthropometric measurements.

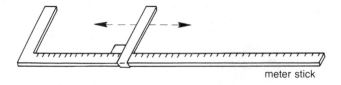

meter stick

FIGURE 7.7   Sliding meter-stick calipers.

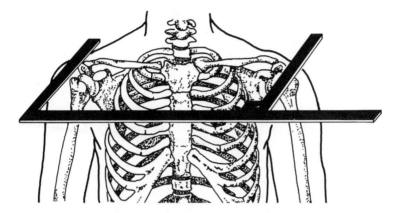

FIGURE 7.8 Shoulder width is the distance between the acromial processes of the shoulder.

Skinfold Measurements. Four sites are measured—the *triceps, biceps, subscapular,* and *supra-iliac* skinfolds.

Equipment and Personnel:

skinfold caliper.

a person to measure and record skinfold.

Procedure for Recorder:

Select the prescribed site and mark it lightly with a felt pen. Grasp the skinfold between the thumb and index finger 1 centimeter above and below the site and apply firm pressure (Figure 7.10). Lift the skinfold, making sure the crest of the fold is aligned as in Figures 7.12–7.15. Apply the caliper jaws at right angles to the prescribed site. Release the spring handles

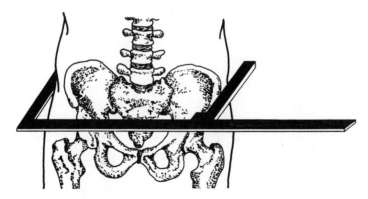

FIGURE 7.9 Hip width is the distance between the two iliac crests.

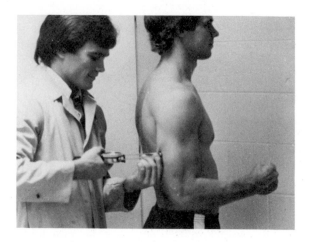

FIGURE 7.10   Position for skinfold measurements.

fully but support the weight of the calipers in your hand (Figure 7.11). Read the measurement after the full pressure of the caliper jaws has been applied and the drift of the needle has ceased. Record to the nearest 0.5 millimeter. Repeat the measurement. If the difference is greater than 2 millimeters, take a third measure and record the mean of the closest pair. Record the readings on score sheet A. Remember that the accuracy of your measurements depends on:

1. precise identification and marking of the site of the skinfold;
2. formation of the skinfold prior to application of the caliper jaws;
3. standardization of the alignment of the skinfold crest;
4. complete release of the spring handles of the caliper.

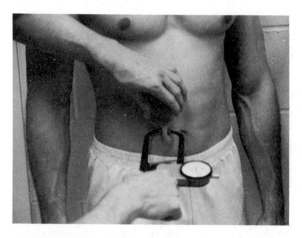

FIGURE 7.11   Skinfold measurements—release grip.

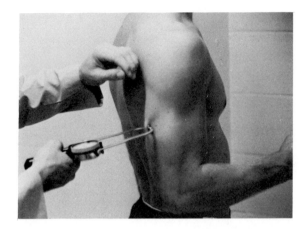

FIGURE 7.12 Triceps skinfold.

Triceps Skinfold. Measure the back of the unclothed pendent right arm at a level midway between the tip of the acromion (Figure 7.12) and the tip of the elbow. With the forearm flexed at an angle of 90 degrees, mark the midpoint with a felt pen. Lift the skinfold parallel to the long axis of the arm. Ask the subject to lower the forearm; then apply the caliper jaws to the site.

Biceps Skinfold. Measure the front of the pendent right upper arm over the biceps, at a level midway between the acromion and the tip of the elbow (as in measuring the triceps skinfold). Lift the skinfold parallel to the long axis of the upper arm (see Figure 7.13).

Subscapular Skinfold. With the subject standing, measure about 1 centimeter below the lower angle of the right scapula. Lift the skinfold so that its crease

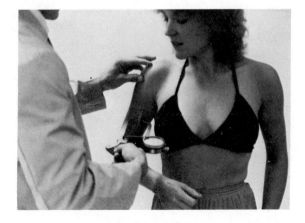

FIGURE 7.13 Biceps skinfold.

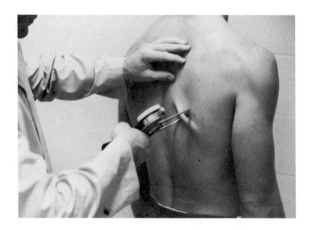

FIGURE 7.14   Subscapular skinfold.

runs at an angle of about 45 degrees downwards from the spine (see Figure 7.14).

Supra-iliac Skinfold.   Measure 3 centimeters above the supra-iliac crest, with the fold running parallel to the crest. (see Figure 7.15).

Percentage of Body Fat Determined From Skinfold Measurements:

1. Determine percentage of body fat: Locate the total of the four skinfold measurements, as recorded on score sheet A, in the leftmost column of Table 7.1 (p. 107). In the appropriate sex and age column of Table 7.1 find the body-fat percentage that corresponds to this total. Record in score sheet A.

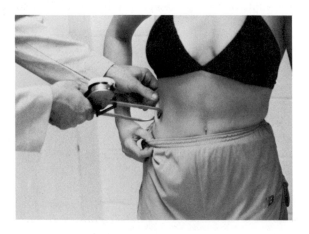

FIGURE 7.15   Supra-iliac skinfold.

2. Evaluate the percentage of body fat: In the appropriate sex and age column of Table 7.2 (p. 108) locate the percentage of body fat. Then find the percentile ranking, in the middle column of the table, that corresponds to this percentage. Record on score sheet A.

3. Determine optimal mass: Use the following formula to calculate your optimal mass (see pp 95–96 for details). Record on score sheet A.

$$\text{Lean body mass (kg.)} = \left[\text{present mass (kg.)} \right.$$

$$\left. - \left(\text{present mass} \times \frac{\% \text{ body fat}}{100} \right) \right]$$

$$= \underline{\hspace{2cm}} \text{ kg. (lean body mass)}$$

Therefore:

$$\text{Optimal mass (kg.)} = \left[\text{lean body mass (kg.)} \right.$$

$$+ \left(\text{lean body mass} \times \frac{\text{desired } \% \text{ body fat}}{100} \right) \right] = \underline{\hspace{2cm}} \text{ kg. (optimal mass)}$$

Percentage of Body Fat Determined From Anthropometric Measurement: *

1. Calculate optimal mass: Find the following 3 anthropometric measurements in score sheet A: height, shoulder (bi-acromial) width, and hip (bi-iliac) width. Then make the following calculations, using these measurements and Table 7.3, and record optimal mass in score sheet A.

The anthropometric measurements from score sheet A must first be converted from centimeters into inches, thus:

$$\text{height (cm.)} \div 2.54 = \underline{\hspace{2cm}} \text{ in.}$$

$$\text{bi-acromial (cm.)} \div 2.54 = \underline{\hspace{2cm}} \text{ in.}$$

$$\text{bi-iliac (cm.)} \div 2.54 = \underline{\hspace{2cm}} \text{ in.}$$

Optimal mass (kg.) = [(a × height) + (b × bi-acromial)+ (c × (bi-iliac) − d] ÷ 2.2

$$= \underline{\hspace{2cm}} \text{ kg.}$$

where: a, b, c, and d are constants obtained from Table 7.3.

* This 3-step procedure and Table 7.3 are adapted from H. B. Falls, A. M. Baylor, and R. K. Dishman, *Essentials of Fitness* (Philadelphia: Saunders College, 1980), pp. 270–272. Reprinted with permission.

TABLE 7.3 Constants for Determining Optimal Mass

	Males			
AGE	CONSTANT a	CONSTANT b	CONSTANT c	CONSTANT d
15–16	0.66	8.27	17.78	217.21
17–19	2.62	10.34	11.24	314.73
20+	1.84	7.10	6.09	145.07
	Females			
AGE	CONSTANT a	CONSTANT b	CONSTANT c	CONSTANT d
15–16	0.84	7.66	15.75	199.14
17–19	1.45	9.28	10.85	207.68
20+	1.12	8.94	9.28	168.01

Note: Since skeletal growth is virtually complete at age 20, the constants for the 20+ age group can be used for all ages above 20.

Source: Adapted from H.B. Falls, A.M. Baylor, and R.K. Dishman. *Essentials of Fitness* (Philadelphia: Saunders College, 1980), p.272. Reprinted with permission.

2. Determine present percentage of body fat and record in score sheet A.

Males: % body fat =

$$\left[\frac{\text{present body mass (kg.)} - (\text{optimal mass (kg.)} \div 1.12)}{\text{present body mass (kg.)}} \right] \times 100$$

Females: % body fat =

$$\left[\frac{\text{present body mass (kg.)} - (\text{optimal mass (kg.)} \div 1.18)}{\text{present body mass (kg.)}} \right] \times 100$$

= _____ %

3. Evaluate percentage of body fat: In the appropriate gender and age column in Table 7.2, locate the percentage of body fat. Then find the percentile ranking, in the middle column of the table, that corresponds to this percentage. Record in score sheet A.

SCORE SHEET A
ANTHROPOMETRIC EVALUATION AND BODY FAT PROFILE

NAME: _____ SEX: _____ AGE: _____ DATE: _____

1. ANTHROPOMETRIC MEASUREMENTS

   Standing Height _____ (cm)

   Body Mass _____ (kg)

   Body Girth Measurements.
     Arm circumference

       Left: _____ (cm)   Right: _____ (cm)

     Chest/Bust circumference: _____ (cm)

     Abdominal circumference: _____ (cm)

     Gluteal circumference: _____ (cm)

     Thigh circumference

       Left: _____ (cm)   Right: _____ (cm)

   Body Width Measurements.

     Shoulder width: _____ (cm)

     Hip width: _____ (cm)

2. BODY FAT DETERMINATION

   Skinfold Measurements.

     Triceps: _____ . ____ (mm)

     Biceps: _____ . ____ (mm)

     Subscapular: _____ . ____ (mm)

     Supra-iliac: _____ . ____ (mm)

       Total: _____ . ____ (mm)

Calculation of % Body Fat and Optimal Mass

From Skinfold Measurements: From Anthropometric Measurements:

   % Body Fat = ____ . ____ %   Optimal Body Mass = _____ . ____ kg

Optimal Body Mass = ____ . ____ kg   % Body Fat = _____ . ____ %
Evaluation of   Evaluation of
   % Body Fat = ____ . ____ % ile*   % Body Fat = _____ . ____ % ile*

*Transfer this score to the Body Fat Profile in the Summary Score Sheet on page 148.

SCORE SHEET B: POSTURE PROFILE EVALUATION

Name _____ Age _____ Sex _____ Date _____

	GOOD - 10	FAIR - 5	POOR - 0		SCORE
HEAD LEFT　　RIGHT	HEAD ERECT GRAVITY LINE PASSES DIRECTLY THROUGH CENTER	HEAD TWISTED OR TURNED TO ONE SIDE SLIGHTLY	HEAD TWISTED OR TURNED TO ONE SIDE MARKEDLY		
SHOULDERS LEFT　　RIGHT	SHOULDERS LEVEL (HORIZONTALLY)	ONE SHOULDER SLIGHTLY HIGHER THAN OTHER	ONE SHOULDER MARKEDLY HIGHER THAN OTHER		
SPINE LEFT　　RIGHT	SPINE STRAIGHT	SPINE SLIGHTLY CURVED LATERALLY	SPINE MARKEDLY CURVED LATERALLY		
HIPS LEFT　　RIGHT	HIPS LEVEL (HORIZONTALLY)	ONE HIP SLIGHTLY HIGHER	ONE HIP MARKEDLY HIGHER		
ANKLES	FEET POINTED STRAIGHT AHEAD	FEET POINTED OUT	FEET POINTED OUT MARKEDLY ANKLES SAG IN (PRONATION)		
NECK	NECK ERECT. CHIN IN, HEAD IN BALANCE DIRECTLY ABOVE SHOULDERS	NECK SLIGHTLY FORWARD, CHIN SLIGHTLY OUT	NECK MARKEDLY FORWARD, CHIN MARKEDLY OUT		
UPPER BACK	UPPER BACK NORMALLY ROUNDED	UPPER BACK SLIGHTLY MORE ROUNDED	UPPER BACK MARKEDLY ROUNDED		
TRUNK	TRUNK ERECT	TRUNK INCLINED TO REAR SLIGHTLY	TRUNK INCLINED TO REAR MARKEDLY		
ABDOMEN	ABDOMEN FLAT	ABDOMEN PROTRUDING	ABDOMEN PROTRUDING AND SAGGING		
LOWER BACK	LOWER BACK NORMALLY CURVED	LOWER BACK SLIGHTLY HOLLOW	LOWER BACK MARKEDLY HOLLOW		
			TOTAL SCORES		/100*

Source: Reproduced through the courtesy of Reedco Research, Auburn, New York.
*Transfer this score to the Posture Profile in the Summary Score Sheet on page 148.

120

B. POSTURE–PROFILE EVALUATION

A single test consisting of 10 separate posture assessments is outlined in score sheet B. Although you can self-administer the test by observing yourself carefully in a full-length mirror, we suggest that you have a colleague (if a specialist is not available) observe your posture and make judgments. The illustrations in score sheet B should be used as a guide. Wear as little clothing as possible when being evaluated. If the evaluation is done in groups, subjects can wear bikini swimsuits.

Score sheet B evaluates ten important areas of posture, from the head to the ankles as well as both anteriorly and posteriorly. Each should be rated on a scale of 0 to 10, and the score placed in the last column of the score sheet. The total score at the bottom of this column indicates your rating out of 100.

C. FLEXIBILITY–PROFILE EVALUATION

The two flexibility tests presented in this section will give you an indication of your level of flexibility in three major regions of the body concerned with fitness: the hips, spine, and shoulders. The first test is the sit-and-reach test, which measures flexion in the sagittal plane at the hip and vertebral joints. The second test measures the flexibility of the shoulder joints and the mobility of the shoulder girdle. Record the results of these tests on score sheet C and then use Tables 7.4 and 7.5 to evaluate them. Finally, average the two evaluation scores to obtain your total flexibility score.

Sit-and-Reach Test

Equipment:
Sit-and-reach apparatus (see Figure 7.16) or modification of same

Procedure:
Before testing, complete a 5-to-10-minute warm-up consisting of slow stretching movements involving the hip and trunk joints (see Chapter 8, phase A). Sit at the apparatus, barefoot and dressed in shorts and T-shirt (or halter top) if required, as shown in Figure 7.17. Holding the legs straight, slowly bend forward with the neck flexed and push the sliding marker with the fingertips as far as possible along the scale. Hold this position for at least 2 seconds. Record the distance and repeat the test. Jerking movements are not permitted, and you must keep the knees straight throughout the test. Record the better of the two measurements on score sheet C. Find the corresponding percentile score in Table 7.4 and record it in score sheet C.

TABLE 7.4 Percentile Scores for Trunk and Hip Flexion (in centimeters)

	Males (age)						PERCENTILE SCORE	Females (age)					
	17–19	20–29	30–39	40–49	50–59	60–65		17–19	20–29	30–39	40–49	50–59	60–65
	59.0	56.0	55.5	54.0	53.0	52.0	100	56.5	56.5	57.0	57.0	55.5	54.0
	46.5	44.5	43.5	42.0	40.5	39.0	95	45.5	45.0	45.5	45.0	44.0	42.5
							Excellent						
	44.5	42.0	41.0	39.5	38.0	36.5	90	43.5	43.0	43.0	42.5	42.0	40.0
	41.5	39.0	38.0	36.5	35.0	33.5	85	41.0	40.5	40.0	39.5	39.0	37.5
	39.5	37.0	36.5	34.5	33.0	31.5	80	39.5	38.5	38.5	37.5	37.5	35.5
	38.0	36.0	35.0	33.0	31.5	30.0	75	38.0	37.0	37.0	36.0	36.0	34.5
	36.5	35.0	33.5	31.5	30.0	28.5	70	37.0	36.0	36.0	35.0	34.5	33.0
	35.5	34.0	32.5	30.5	28.5	27.0	65	36.0	35.0	35.0	33.5	33.5	32.0
	34.0	32.5	31.0	29.0	27.5	26.0	60	35.0	34.0	33.5	32.5	32.5	31.0
	33.0	31.5	30.0	28.0	26.0	24.5	55	34.0	33.0	32.5	31.5	31.5	30.0
							Average						
	32.0	30.5	29.0	27.0	25.0	23.5	50	33.0	32.0	31.5	30.0	30.0	28.5
	30.5	29.5	28.0	26.0	24.0	22.0	45	32.0	31.0	30.0	29.0	29.0	27.5
	29.5	28.5	27.0	25.0	22.5	21.0	40	31.0	30.0	29.0	28.0	28.0	26.5
	28.0	27.0	25.5	23.5	21.5	19.5	35	30.0	28.5	28.0	26.5	27.0	24.5
	27.0	26.0	24.5	22.5	20.0	18.5	30	29.0	27.5	27.0	25.5	26.0	24.5
	25.5	25.0	23.1	21.0	18.5	17.0	25	27.5	26.0	26.0	24.5	24.5	23.0
	24.0	23.5	21.5	19.5	17.0	15.5	20	26.0	25.0	24.0	22.5	23.0	21.5
	22.5	21.5	20.0	17.5	15.0	13.5	15	24.5	23.0	22.5	21.0	21.5	20.0
	19.0	19.0	17.0	14.5	12.0	10.5	10	22.0	20.5	20.0	18.0	18.5	17.0
	17.0	16.5	14.5	12.5	9.5	8.0	5	20.0	18.0	17.5	16.5	16.5	15.0
	5.0	5.0	2.5	0.0	0.0	0.0	0	9.5	7.0	6.0	5.5	5.0	3.5

TABLE 7.5   Ratings for Shoulder-Girdle Flexibility

RATING (/100)	X̄ Distance Between Thumbs (centimeters)	
	MALES	FEMALES
100	0	0
Excellent		
90	2	1
80	4	3
70	6	5
60	8	7
Average		
50	10	9
40	12	11
30	14	13
20	16	15
10	18	17
0	20	19

These ratings are unrelated to age.

Shoulder-Flexibility Test

Equipment and Personnel:
measuring tape
tester

Procedure for Tester:
The subject should be shirtless or dressed in a halter top.

Before testing, a 1-to-2-minute warm-up involving slow, controlled forward and backward full arm circles should be performed (see Chapter 8, phase A). Have the subject stand with his or her back to you and attempt to touch the ends of the thumbs behind the back (Figure 7.18). The left hand reaches over the shoulder, behind and below the head, while the right hand is placed on the back in the lumbar region and then raised. Measure the

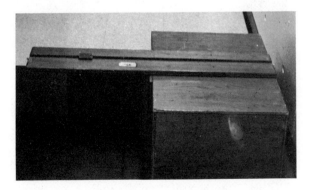

FIGURE 7.16   Sit-and-reach apparatus.

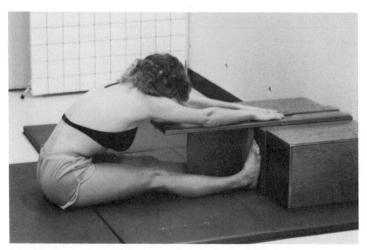

FIGURE 7.17   Measurement of trunk and hip flexion.

distance between the thumbs. The hand and arm positions are reversed for the second measurement (right hand over the shoulder). Record both measurements on score sheet C and calculate their average. Find the corresponding rating in Table 7.5 and record it on the score sheet. If the thumbs touch in both measurements, award the maximum rating of 100.

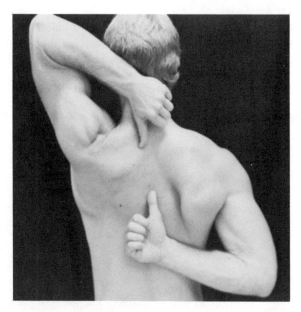

FIGURE 7.18   Shoulder flexibility test.

SCORE SHEET C
FLEXIBILITY-PROFILE EVALUATION

NAME _____ SEX _____ AGE _____ DATE _____

Sit-and-reach-test

    trial 1 _____ cm.

    trial 2 _____ cm.

    evaluation of hip and trunk flexibility _____ %ile

Shoulder-flexibility test

        left over right _____ cm.

        right over left _____ cm.

    mean distance apart _____ cm.

    evaluation of shoulder mobility _____ /100

        mean flexibility score [*]

*Transfer this score to the Summary Score Sheet on page 148.

D. MUSCULAR PROFILE: ENDURANCE AND STRENGTH

This section consists of five tests of muscular endurance and muscular strength. Both males and females can perform these tests. It is not necessary to perform all the tests in order to establish your muscular profile. As we noted in Chapter 4, muscular endurance is considered a more important indicator of physical fitness than muscular strength. None of the muscular-endurance tests requires specialized equipment, and all can be performed by younger, more active persons. Older and less active people should be aware of the strenuous demands of the tests when correctly performed. Moreover, the One-minute sit-up test should not be performed by those who are predisposed to lower-back pain. The muscular-strength tests require equipment usually found in exercise laboratories and fitness centers. Record all test scores and the corresponding percentile rankings from Tables 7.6–7.10, on score sheet D. Finally, average the five rankings to determine a mean rating of your muscular endurance and strength.

TABLE 7.6 Percentile Scores for Number of Sit-Ups Completed in 1 Minute

	Males (age)						PERCENTILE SCORE	Females (age)					
	17–19	20–29	30–39	40–49	50–59	60–65		17–19	20–29	30–39	40–49	50–59	60–65
	63	61	53	47	42	43	100	56	51	42	37	32	31
	52	49	43	37	32	31	95	44	40	32	28	23	22
							Excellent						
	50	47	40	35	30	29	90	42	37	30	26	21	20
	48	44	38	32	28	27	85	39	35	27	23	19	18
	46	42	36	31	26	25	80	37	33	26	22	18	17
	45	41	35	30	25	24	75	36	31	25	21	17	16
	43	40	34	28	24	22	70	34	30	24	20	16	15
	42	38	33	27	23	21	65	33	29	23	19	15	14
	41	37	31	26	22	20	60	32	28	22	18	14	13
	40	36	30	25	21	19	55	31	27	21	17	13	12
							Average						
	39	35	29	25	20	18	50	30	26	20	16	12	11
	38	34	28	24	19	17	45	29	25	19	15	11	10
	37	33	27	23	18	16	40	27	24	18	14	11	9
	36	32	26	22	17	15	35	26	23	17	13	10	8
	35	31	25	21	16	14	30	25	21	16	12	9	7
	34	29	24	19	15	13	25	24	20	15	11	8	6
	32	28	23	18	14	11	20	22	19	13	10	7	5
	31	26	21	17	12	10	15	20	17	12	8	5	4
	28	23	18	14	10	7	10	17	14	9	6	3	2
	20	21	16	12	8	5	5	15	12	7	4	2	1
	15	9	5	2	0	0	0	3	1	0	0	0	0

TABLE 7.7 Percentile Scores for Number of Push-Ups Completed

Males (age)						PERCENTILE SCORE	Females (age)					
17–19	20–29	30–39	40–49	50–59	60–65		17–19	20–29	30–39	40–49	50–59	60–65
65	56	48	41	37	37	100	45	44	46	38	32	29
49	41	35	29	26	25	95	32	32	32	27	22	20
						Excellent						
45	39	33	27	24	23	90	31	30	29	24	20	18
41	35	29	25	22	20	85	28	26	26	22	18	16
38	33	27	23	20	19	80	26	25	24	20	17	15
36	31	26	22	19	17	75	25	23	22	19	15	14
34	29	24	20	17	16	70	23	22	21	17	14	13
32	28	23	19	16	15	65	22	21	20	16	13	12
31	26	22	18	15	14	60	21	19	18	15	12	11
29	25	21	17	14	13	55	20	18	17	14	12	10
						Average						
27	23	19	16	13	12	50	19	17	16	13	11	9
26	22	18	15	12	10	45	17	16	14	12	10	8
24	21	17	14	11	9	40	16	15	13	11	9	7
22	19	16	13	10	8	35	15	14	12	10	8	6
21	18	14	12	9	7	30	14	12	10	9	7	5
19	16	13	11	8	6	25	13	11	9	7	6	4
16	14	11	9	7	4	20	11	9	7	6	5	3
14	12	9	7	5	3	15	9	8	5	4	3	2
9	8	6	5	2	1	10	6	5	2	2	1	1
6	6	4	3	1	0	5	4	2	1	1	0	0
0	0	0	0	0	0	0	0	0	0	0	0	0

TABLE 7.8 Percentile Scores for
Number of Chin-Ups
Completed

PERCENTILE SCORE	MALES	FEMALES
100	10	5
Excellent		
90	9	4.5
80	8	4
70	7	3.5
60	6	3
Average		
50	5	2.5
40	4	2
30	3	1.5
20	2	1
10	1	0.5
0	0	0

These percentile scores are unrelated to age.

1. Muscular–Endurance Tests

The following three tests require little equipment and use your own body mass as the resistance: One-Minute Speed Sit-Ups, Push-Ups, and Chin-Ups.

One-Minute Sit-Up Test

Equipment and Personnel:
mat
timer

Procedure for Timer:
Have the subject lie supine, knees bent at a right angle and the feet 30 centimeters apart. The hands with fingers interlocked are placed behind the head, and must be maintained in this position for the duration of the test (Figure 7.19a). Hold the subject's ankles so that the heels are kept in contact with the mat. For each sit-up the elbows must touch the knees as shown in Figure 7.19b. When ready, give the command "Begin." The subject must sit up and touch the knees with the elbows and return to the starting position.

The subject performs as many repetitions as possible within one minute. The subject may pause whenever necessary.

Ensure that the interlocked fingers make contact with the mat when the subject returns to the starting position. The subject should exhale when sitting up. Record the number of sit-ups completed in 60 seconds on score sheet D.

TABLE 7.9 Percentile Scores for Hand-Grip Strength (in Kilograms)

Males (age)						PERCENTILE SCORE	Females (age)					
17–19	20–29	30–39	40–49	50–59	60–65		17–19	20–29	30–39	40–49	50–59	60–65
138	142	143	140	131	123	100	94	83	84	86	78	71
117	121	122	119	111	105	95	75	70	70	71	65	59
						Excellent						
113	117	118	115	107	101	90	72	67	68	68	63	56
107	112	113	110	102	96	85	67	63	64	64	59	53
104	109	110	107	99	93	80	64	61	62	62	58	52
102	106	107	104	97	91	75	62	60	61	60	56	50
99	104	105	102	95	89	70	60	58	59	58	54	49
97	102	103	100	93	87	65	58	57	58	57	53	47
95	100	101	98	91	85	60	56	55	56	55	52	46
93	98	99	96	89	84	55	55	54	55	54	51	45
						Average						
91	96	97	94	87	82	50	53	53	54	52	50	44
89	94	95	92	85	80	45	51	52	53	51	48	43
87	92	93	90	83	78	40	50	50	51	49	47	42
85	90	91	88	81	76	35	48	49	50	48	46	41
83	88	89	86	79	75	30	46	48	49	46	45	40
81	86	87	84	77	72	25	44	46	47	45	44	38
78	83	84	81	75	70	20	41	44	45	43	41	37
75	80	81	78	72	67	15	39	42	43	40	40	35
69	75	76	73	67	63	10	34	39	40	36	36	32
65	71	72	69	63	59	5	31	36	37	33	34	30
44	50	51	48	43	40	0	12	22	24	18	21	18

TABLE 7.10 Percentile Scores For Leg-Lift Strength (in Kilograms)

Males (age)		PERCENTILE SCORE	Females (age)	
17–25	26–45		17–25	26–45
380	356	100	162	136
365	342	95	156	131
		excellent		
349	328	90	150	126
334	313	85	145	121
318	299	80	139	116
303	285	75	133	111
287	270	70	127	106
272	256	65	122	101
256	241	60	115	96
241	227	55	109	91
		average		
225	213	50	103	86
210	198	45	97	81
195	184	40	91	76
179	170	35	85	71
164	155	30	80	66
148	141	25	74	61
133	127	20	68	56
117	113	15	62	51
102	98	10	56	46
86	83	5	50	41
71	69	0	45	36

Source: Adapted from M. S. Yuhasz, *Physical Fitness Appraisal* (London, Ontario: Unversity of Western Ontario, 1982), pp. 21–24. Reprinted by permission.

Push-Up Test

Equipment and Personnel:
flat surface such as a mat or carpet
counter

Procedure (Males):
Lie on your front, legs together. Point the hands forward and position them under the shoulders. (See Figure 7.20a.) Push up from the mat by straightening the elbows and using the toes as pivots (Figure 7.20b). Keep the upper body rigid and in a straight line. Then return to the starting position, chin to the mat.

Procedure (Females):
Lie on your front, legs together. Hands pointing forward are positioned under the shoulders. Push up from the mat by straightening the elbows

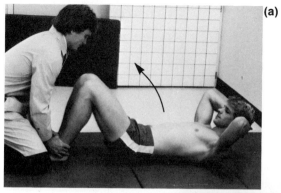
(a)

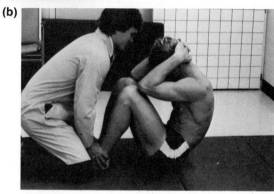
(b)

FIGURE 7.19 One-minute sit-up test: (a) starting position; (b) elbows must touch knees in each sit-up.

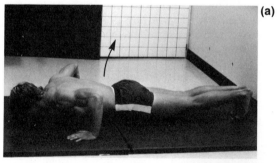
(a)

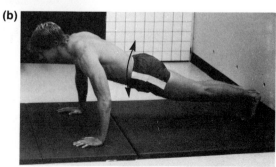
(b)

FIGURE 7.20 Push-up test for males.

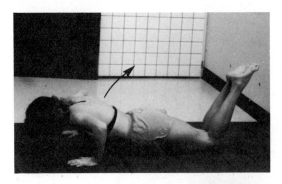

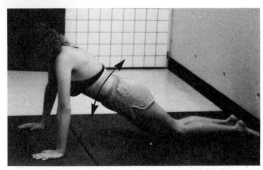

FIGURE 7.21 Push-up test for females.

and using the knees as pivots (Figure 7.21a). Keep the upper body rigid and in a straight line. Then return to the starting position, chin to the mat, and allow the feet to swing upwards simultaneously (Figure 7.21b).

Procedure for Counter:

The push-ups are to be performed consecutively and without a time limit. Discontinue the test as soon as you see the subject strain forcibly to complete a push-up. Count the initial push-up and each repetition successfully completed. Record the score on score sheet D.

Chin-Up Test

Equipment:

a sturdy bar suspended above a standing person's outstretched hands

Procedure:

Hang from the bar with hands in undergrip position (Figure 7.22a). Flex elbows and extend shoulder joints (Figure 7.22b) to lift the body so that the chin passes over the level of the bar. Then lower the body so that both arms are straight again. Repeat as many times as possible. Record the number of chin-ups completed, to the nearest half chin-up (i.e., when elbow flexion reaches 90 degrees), on score sheet D.

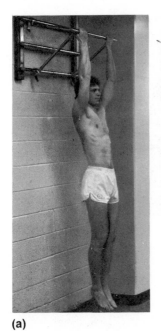 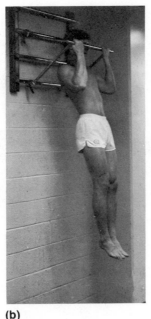

FIGURE 7.22 Chin-up test.

(a)   **(b)**

2. Muscular–Strength Tests

Included in the tests of muscular strength are two assessments which require testing equipment: the test of grip strength requires a hand dynamometer and the knee extension test requires a leg dynamometer.

Hand-Grip Test

Equipment:
an accurate hand-grip dynamometer

Procedure:
Adjust the grip of the dynamometer to the size of the left hand; find the most comfortable setting. The second joint of the fingers should fit comfortably under the handle and take the weight of the instrument. Hold the grip between the fingers and the palm at the base of the thumb, as shown in Figure 7.23. Hold the instrument away from the body and squeeze with maximum force. Neither the hand nor the dynamometer is allowed to touch the body or any other object. Now measure the right hand. Conclude with a second trial for each hand. Add the best score for the left hand to the best score for the right hand and record as a single score, to the nearest kilogram, on score sheet D.

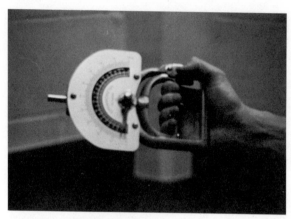

FIGURE 7.23 Hand grip.

Leg-Lift Strength Test

> *Equipment and Personnel:*
> tester
> belt
> a leg dynamometer—a scale mounted on a platform, with an adjustable chain, and a metal bar (the handle) attached; the scale measures from 0 to 1000 kilograms, and its dial has an indicator needle that remains in place after a maximum effort by the subject

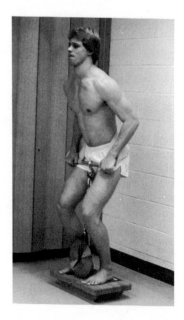

FIGURE 7.24
Leg-lift strength test.

SCORE SHEET D
MUSCULAR PROFILE: ENDURANCE AND STRENGTH

NAME _____ SEX _____ AGE _____ DATE _____

1. Muscular-endurance tests

	test score		rating
1-minute sit-ups	_____ (no.)		_____%ile
push-ups	_____ (no.)		_____%ile
chin-ups	_____ (no.)		_____%ile

2. Muscular-strength tests

hand-grip test (left and right)	_____ kg.		_____%ile
leg-lift test	_____ kg.		_____%ile
mean rating of muscular endurance and strength			*

*Transfer this score to the Summary Score Sheet on page 148.

Procedure for Tester:

Have the subject stand erect on the platform of the dynamometer, back and buttocks flat against a wall, and then lower the body until the knees are flexed at approximately 55 degrees (see Figure 7.24). Adjust the chain length so that the bar rests at the top of the thighs along the bend of the waist on foam padding. Then secure the bar to the subject's waist with the belt, circling it tightly around the waist and fixing both ends of it to the bar (Figure 7.24). Instruct the subject to gradually lift straight up by extending the legs. Help the subject keep back and buttocks against the wall. Conduct two more trials, and record the best of the three, to the nearest 2 kilograms, on score sheet D.

E. AEROBIC–FITNESS PROFILE

The four standardized tests in this section were selected because of their range of application (see Table 7.11). The first three tests *predict* aerobic fitness; the fourth is the standard laboratory test for directly measuring maximal oxygen consumption. The first and third tests require little equipment, whereas the other two are performed in a laboratory. Two tests employ only submaximal (light

TABLE 7.11   Four Standardized Tests for Evaluating Aerobic Fitness

TECHNICAL EQUIPMENT	EXERCISE INTENSITY	
	SUBMAXIMAL	MAXIMAL
not required	1. Step test* (Bench 50.8 cm. high)	3. 12-minute run* (400-meter track)
required	2. Astrand-Rhyming test* (bicycle ergometer)	4. Balke test (treadmill and gas spirometry)

Before taking any of these tests, especially the maximal tests, consult your doctor.
*These three tests predict aerobic fitness; the Balke test is a direct measure of maximal oxygen consumption.

to moderate) exercise and monitor your physiological response (as measured by your heart rate). These tests should be selected by older or unfit persons. The other two tests employ maximal exercise (exercise carried out to the point of exhaustion). To evaluate your aerobic fitness, *you need complete only one of the four tests.* You may, however, perform two (or more) and then enter the best test result in your Summmary Score Sheet, p. 148.

Tests Employing Submaximal Exercise

Test 1: 3-Minute Step Test

Equipment:
A bench, heavy chair, or similar platform, 50.8 cm (20 in.) high
A watch or clock with a sweep second hand

Procedure:
Step UP. . .UP. . . onto the bench, first with the right foot, then with the left.
Then step DOWN. . .DOWN. . . from the bench back down to the floor, first with the right foot, then with the left. Continue the sequence in rhythm, stepping UP. . .UP. . .DOWN. . .DOWN. . . at a rate of 30 steps per minute, or one complete UP-and-DOWN every 2 seconds, as illustrated in Figure 7.25.
After 3 minutes, or 90 complete repetitions, immediately sit down on the bench and remain sitting quietly for three and one-half minutes. During this recovery period you will periodically count your pulse (by palpitation of the radial artery at the wrist) as follows:

1. After 1 minute of recovery count your pulse for 30 seconds.
2. After 2 minutes of recovery count your pulse for another 30 seconds.
3. After 3 minutes of recovery make a final 30-second pulse count.

Record each of these three pulse counts in score sheet E.1 and add them up. Then find the corresponding percentile ranking from Table 7.12.

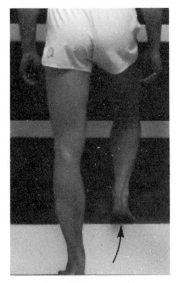

(a) Step UP with right foot. [0:00.5 sec.]

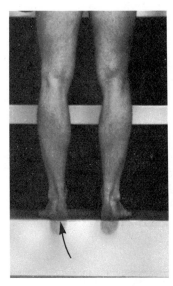

(b) Bring UP the left and stand erect. [0:01.0 sec.]

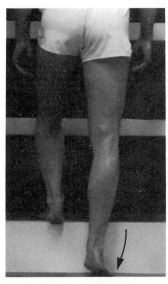

(c) Step DOWN with the right. [0:01.5 sec.]

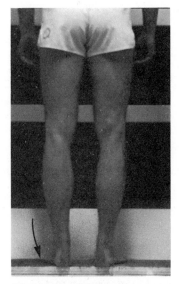

(d) Bring the left foot DOWN. [0:02.0 sec.]

FIGURE 7.25 Performing a step test using a bench. Elapsed time is shown in brackets. Each complete sequence takes 2 seconds.

TABLE 7.12 Percentile Scores for 3-Minute Step Test

Males (Age)		PERCENTILE	Females (Age)	
17–25	26–50	SCORE	17–25	26–50
108	110	100	122	125
115	117	95	128	131
		Excellent		
121	123	90	134	137
128	130	85	140	143
134	136	80	146	149
141	142	75	153	155
147	149	70	158	161
154	155	65	165	167
160	162	60	170	173
167	168	55	177	179
		Average		
173	174	50	183	185
180	181	45	189	191
186	187	40	195	197
193	193	35	212	213
199	200	30	217	219
206	206	25	224	225
212	213	20	229	231
219	219	15	236	237
225	225	10	242	243
232	232	5	249	249
238	238	0	256	256

Source: Adapted from M.S. Yuhasz, *Physical Fitness Appraisal* (London, Ontario: University of Western Ontario, 1982), pp. 26–27. Reprinted by permission.

Test 2: Astrand-Rhyming Bicycle Ergometer Test[3]

Equipment:

mechanically braked bicycle ergometer

metronome (set so that a person following its beat will be pedaling at 50 revolutions per minute)

Optional Equipment:

3-lead electrocardiogram for recording heart rate

Directions:

1. Set the work load of the bicycle ergometer so that your target heart rate while pedaling at 50 revolutions per minute will be between 140 and 160 beats per minute. (The work load setting is usually between 450 and 900 kilogram-meters and depends on the level of aerobic fitness, age, sex, etc., of the subject.)

SCORE SHEET E.1
AEROBIC-FITNESS PROFILE

NAME _____ SEX _____ AGE _____ DATE _____

Test 1: 3-minute step test

Heart rates	
Recording period	Number of pulses counted
$1-1^1/_2$ minutes postexercise:	_____
$2-2^1/2$ minutes postexercise:	_____
$3-3^1/_2$ minutes postexercise:	_____
sum of the 3 pulse counts:	_____

evaluation of 3-minute step test

percentile score (from Table 7.12): _____%ile*

*Transfer this score to the Summary Score Sheet, page 148.

---

2. Pedal for 6 minutes, counting your heart rate by palpitation (or by EKG) over the last 15 seconds of each minute. (Then multiplied by 4 to obtain the number of beats per minute.) After the second or third minute, you may have to adjust the ergometer work load so that the target heart rate (140 to 160 beats per minute) is achieved.
3. Over the final 3 minutes of this 6-minute test your heart rate should remain constant, between 140 and 160 beats per minute. This average, steady heart rate is used to predict aerobic fitness. Record the heart rates, in beats per minute, in score sheet E.2. Then use Figure 7.26 to determine your predicted maximal oxygen consumption. Finally find the corresponding percentile ranking in Table 7.13.

Tests Employing Maximal Exercise

Test 3: 12-Minute Run

Equipment and Personnel:
outdoor 400-meter track or indoor track with 100-meter distances marked
watch with a sweep second hand
timer

SCORE SHEET E.2
AEROBIC-FITNESS PROFILE

NAME _____ SEX _____ AGE _____ DATE _____

Test 2: Astrand-Rhyming Test

_____ Heart rates _____

time (min.)	bicycle ergometer work load (kg.)	heart rate (beats/min.)
1	_____	_____
2	_____	_____
3	_____	_____
4	_____	_____
5	_____	_____
6	_____	_____

Should be relatively constant, between 140 and 160 beats per minute. Determine the average heart rate for this 3-minute period; this value will be utilized in Figure 7.26.

Predicted maximal oxygen consumption (from Figure 7.26)

maximal O_2 consumption = _____ liters/min.
maximal O_2 consumption in terms of body mass

$$= \left[\frac{\text{max. } O_2 \text{ consumption (liters/min.)}}{\text{body mass (kg.)}} \right] \times 1000$$

$$= \text{_____ milliliters } O_2/\text{kg./min.}$$

Evaluation of predicted maximal O_2 *consumption*

percentile score (from Table 7.13)   _____ %ile*

*Transfer this score to the Summary Score Sheet on page 148.

Procedure for timer:

After giving the command to begin, count the number of laps of the track completed. At the end of 12 minutes, determine the completed distance around the final lap, to the nearest ten meters.

Procedure for Subject:

1. Following a thorough warm-up, run as far as possible in 12 minutes. At the end of 12 minutes you *must be exhausted* in order for the test to give a valid prediction of aerobic capacity. (To achieve complete exhaustion in 12 minutes, perform the test 2 or 3 times to ensure that you run as far as possible in the time limit.)

2. Calculate your predicted maximal oxygen consumption in score sheet E.3.

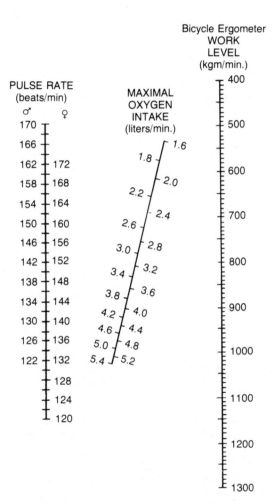

FIGURE 7.26 Prediction of aerobic fitness by submaximal exercise on the bicycle ergometer. Locate your pulse rate in the male (♂) or female (♀) scale on the left. On the right-hand scale locate your bicycle ergometer work load. Draw a straight line connecting the two points. Where this line intersects the middle scale is the reading of your predicted maximal oxygen consumption. *Source*: Adapted from P.-O. Astrand and I. Rhyming, "A Nomogram for Calculation of Aerobic Capacity (Physical Fitness) from Pulse Rate during Submaximal Work," *Journal of Applied Physiology*, 7 (1954) 218-221.

TABLE 7.13 Percentile Scores for Predicted Maximal Oxygen Consumption (in millimeters O_2/kg./min.)

Males (age)						PERCENTILE SCORE	Females (age)					
17–19	20–29	30–39	40–49	50–59	60–65		17–19	20–29	30–39	40–49	50–59	60–65
67.9	63.1	54.0	47.4	43.8	40.1	100	46.2	44.5	41.6	38.7	36.3	32.1
60.8	56.2	48.7	42.9	39.2	35.6	95	42.7	40.5	37.7	34.5	31.2	27.8
59.4	54.9	47.6	42.0	38.3	34.7	90 Excellent	42.0	39.7	37.0	33.7	30.2	27.0
57.7	53.2	46.3	40.9	37.2	33.6	85	41.1	38.7	36.0	32.6	28.9	25.9
56.6	52.2	45.5	40.3	36.5	32.9	80	40.6	38.1	35.5	32.0	28.2	25.3
55.7	51.4	44.8	39.7	35.9	32.3	75	40.2	37.7	35.0	31.5	27.6	24.8
54.9	50.6	44.3	39.2	35.4	31.8	70	39.8	37.2	34.5	31.0	27.0	24.3
54.3	50.0	43.7	38.8	35.0	31.4	65	39.4	36.8	34.2	30.6	26.5	23.9
53.5	49.3	43.2	38.3	34.5	30.9	60	39.0	36.4	33.8	30.2	26.0	23.4
52.9	48.7	42.7	37.9	34.1	30.5	55 Average	38.8	36.1	33.4	29.8	25.5	23.1
52.2	48.0	42.2	37.5	33.6	30.1	50	38.3	35.7	33.1	29.4	25.0	22.6
51.5	47.4	41.7	37.0	33.2	29.6	45	38.1	35.3	32.7	29.0	24.6	22.2
50.9	46.8	41.2	36.6	32.8	29.2	40	37.7	35.0	32.4	28.7	24.1	21.9
50.2	46.1	40.7	36.2	32.3	28.7	35	37.4	34.6	32.0	28.2	23.6	21.4
49.5	45.4	40.2	35.8	31.9	28.3	30	37.0	34.2	31.6	27.8	23.1	21.0
48.7	44.7	39.6	35.3	31.4	27.8	25	36.6	33.8	31.2	27.4	22.5	20.5
47.8	43.8	38.9	34.7	30.8	27.2	20	36.2	33.3	30.7	26.8	21.9	20.0
46.7	42.8	38.1	34.0	30.1	26.6	15	35.7	32.7	30.1	26.2	21.1	19.4
45.0	41.1	36.8	32.9	29.0	25.4	10	34.8	31.7	29.1	25.2	19.9	18.3
43.6	39.8	35.8	32.0	28.1	24.5	5	34.1	30.9	28.4	24.4	18.9	17.5
36.5	33.0	20.4	27.5	23.5	20.0	0	30.6	27.0	24.5	20.2	13.8	13.2

SCORE SHEET E.3
AEROBIC-FITNESS PROFILE

NAME _____ SEX _____ AGE _____ DATE _____

Test 3: 12-minute run test

Total distance run:

$$\left[\underline{\hspace{3cm}} \times \underline{\hspace{2cm}} \right] + \underline{\hspace{3cm}} = \underline{\hspace{2cm}} \text{ meters}$$

distance of 1 lap no. of laps   completed distance   total distance run
of track (in m.)   completed   of final lap (m.)

Average speed of running:

$$\underline{\hspace{3cm}} \text{(m.)} \div 12 \text{ minutes} = \underline{\hspace{3cm}} \text{ m./min.}$$

total distance run   average speed of running

Predicted maximal O_2 consumption:

$$33.3 \text{ ml. } O_2/\text{kg.}/\text{m.} + \left[\underline{\hspace{2cm}} \text{ m./min.} - 150 \text{ m./min.} \right] \times 0.21 =$$

average speed

$$\underline{\hspace{4cm}} \text{ ml. } O_2/\text{kg.}/\text{min.}$$

predicted max. O_2 consumption

where: 33.3 ml. O_2/kg./min. is the O_2 requirement for running at 150 m./min.
0.21 ml O_2/kg./min. is the O_2 cost of running each m./min. faster than
150 m./min.

Evaluation of 12-minute run test

percentile score (from Table 7.13) _____%ile*

*Transfer this score to the Summary Score Sheet on page 148.

Test 4. Balke Maximal Oxygen Consumption Test[4].

Equipment and Personnel:

motor-driven treadmill

open-circuit gas-collection system (Figure 7.27)

3-way breathing valve, mouthpiece, nose clip and headgear support (for
breathing valve)

wide-bore Collins tubing

On the inspired-gas line: gasometer for measuring the volume of inspired
air (in liters)

On the expired-gas line: mixing chamber when 0_2 and CO_2 analyzers connected downstream by small-bore plastic tubing

3- or 4-lead electrocardiogram and recorder

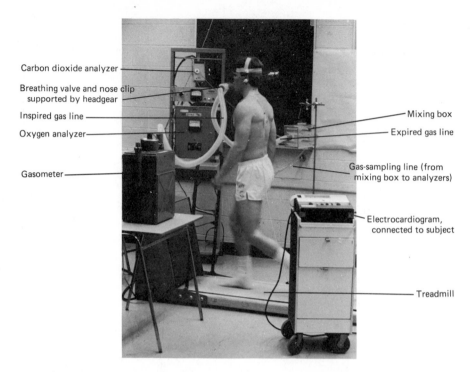

Carbon dioxide analyzer

Breathing valve and nose clip
supported by headgear

Inspired gas line

Oxygen analyzer

Gasometer

Mixing box

Expired gas line

Gas-sampling line (from
mixing box to analyzers)

Electrocardiogram,
connected to subject

Treadmill

FIGURE 7.27 Subject walking on a treadmill during the Balke Maximal Oxygen Consumption Test, breathing through the open-circuit gas-collection system. Room air is inspired through the inspired-gas line connected to a gasometer, which measures gas volume in liters per minute. The subject's expired air is directed by the breathing valve through the expired-gas line into the mixing box, where small samples of expired air are continuously drawn into the oxygen and carbon dioxide analyzers. Heart rate can also be monitored periodically during the test by a 3- or 4-lead electrocardiogram.

Procedure for Subject:

1. Stand quietly on the treadmill for 5 to 10 minutes so that your resting oxygen consumption, ventilation, and heart rate can be determined.

2. Following this preexercise period, begin walking on the treadmill—at 80 meters per minute (3.0 mph) for females and 90.7 meters per minute (3.4 mph) for males—until you are exhausted.

3. You can predict your maximal oxygen consumption from Table 7.14 or calculate it directly in score sheet E.4. Then find the corresponding percentile score in Table 7.13 in order to predict your aerobic fitness.

Procedure for Tester:

1. Raise the treadmill grade at set intervals, as follows: The subject walks at a 0-percent grade for the first 3 minutes. Then raise the treadmill to a 5 percent grade for the next 3 minutes, and to a 10 percent grade for the 3 minutes after that. Thereafter raise the treadmill grade 2.5 percent every 2.5 minutes until the subject is exhausted (unable to continue to the next grade).

TABLE 7.14   Predicting Maximal O_2 Consumption From the Speed and Final Slope of the Treadmill

Treadmill Slope at Exhaustion (%)	Predicted O_2 Consumption (ml. O_2/kg./min.)	
	FEMALES	MALES
2.5	10.3	17.7
5.0	14.1	21.5
7.5	17.3	24.7
10.0	21.1	28.5
12.5	24.4	31.8
15.0	28.4	35.8
.17.5	31.5	38.7
20.0	35.7	43.1
22.5	38.1	45.5
25.0	41.9	49.3
27.5	44.7	52.1
30.0	48.2	55.6

Source: B. Balke and R. W. Ware, "An Experimental Study of 'Physical Fitness' of Air Force Personnel," *United States Armed Forces Medical Journal,* 10 (1959), 675–88.

2. Measure the subject's ventilation, oxygen consumption, and heart rate while he or she is at a standing rest; (a) over a 1-minute period preexercise, and (b) over the last full minute of each work load (grade).

3. You may skip data collection at some of the lower grades. However, above a heart rate of 160 or 170 beats per minute, the subject will only have a few more work loads left; therefore carefully determine all data over the last minute of each subsequent work load up to the exhaustion work load (the final grade that the subject can complete). Record all data on score sheet E.4.

SUMMARY: PERSONAL FITNESS RATING AND EVALUATION

In this final section we first help you determine your personal fitness rating. We then outline a sequence of steps by which you can evaluate your testing results from this chapter.

Determination of Your Personal Fitness Rating

First, in the upper half of the summary score sheet fill in your ratings from the five individual profile areas in the spaces provided at the bottom of each thermometer. These ratings are the percentile scores (percentage score in the case of the posture profile) that you determined at the end of each profile (each was marked with an asterisk). Then, for all profiles in which your score

SCORE SHEET E.4
AEROBIC FITNESS PROFILE

NAME _____ SEX _____ AGE _____ DATE _____

Test 4: Balke treadmill test: physiological and oxygen consumption data

1. Predicted maximal O_2 consumption
   From the speed of the treadmill and the final treadmill slope at exhaustion, predict maximal O_2 consumption according to Table 7.14: _____ ml. O_2/kg./min.*

2. Direct determination of maximal O_2 consumption
   a. Record the following data:

   height: _____·_____ cm.   mass: _____·_____ kg.   laboratory temp: _____·_____°C

   STPD factor: 0.9 ____ ____
   b. Record the data obtained throughout the Balke test:

Slope of tm (%)	Heart rate (/min.)	Inspired ventilation (l./min., STPD)†	Expired O₂ (%)	CO₂ (%)	O₂ consumption† (l./min., STPD)	(ml./kg./min.)**
pre-exercise	____	____	__	__	____	_____
0	____	____	__	__	____	_____
5	____	____	__	__	____	_____
10	____	____	__	__	____	_____
12.5	____	____	__	__	____	_____
15.0	____	____	__	__	____	_____
17.5	____	____	__	__	____	_____
20.0	____	____	__	__	____	_____
22.5	____	____	__	__	____	_____
25.0	____	____	__	__	____	_____
27.5	____	____	__	__	____	_____
30.0	____	____	__	__	____	_____
____	____	____	__	__	____	_____

c. Calculate maximal O_2 consumption:
Oxygen consumption ($\dot{V}O_2$) can be calculated according to the following formula:

$$\dot{V}O_2 = \dot{V}_I \times F_{IO_2} \quad - \quad \dot{V}_E \times F_{EO_2}$$

where: $\dot{V}O_2$ = O_2 consumption in liters O_2/minute STPD
$\dot{V}_I$ = inspired ventilation, in l./min. STPD
($\dot{V}_I$ = measured inspired volume of air over one minute $\times$ STPD factor; the STPD factor is approximately 0.9 at normal laboratory temperatures [18 to 22° C] at sea level)

F_{IO_2} = fraction of oxygen in the inspired air; assumed to be 0.2093 (i.e., the percentage of inspired oxygen is 20.93)

$$\dot{V}_E = \dot{V}_I \text{ (l./min. STPD)} \times \frac{79.04}{100 - (F_{EO_2} + F_{ECO_2})}$$

F_{ECO_2} ranges between 0.035 and 0.055; i.e., the percentage of expired carbon dioxide is between 3.5 and 5.5)

F_{EO_2} = fraction of oxygen in the expired air; ranges between 0.145 to 0.170 (i.e., the percentage of expired oxygen is between 14.5 and 17.5)

Oxygen consumption ($\dot{V}O_2$) is converted from liters O_2 per minute to milliliters O_2/kg./min. by the following formula:

$$\dot{V}O_2 \text{(ml. } O_2\text{/kg./min.)} = \left[\frac{\dot{V}O_2 \text{(l/min)} \times 1000}{\text{body mass (kg.)}} \right]$$

*Use this value to find your aerobic-fitness score in Table 7.13. Then transfer that percentile score to the Summary Score Sheet, p. 148.

†The formula for determining inspired ventilation and O_2 consumption, in liters per minute STPD, is explained above.

**Use the final value in this column (the exhaustion work load) to find your aerobic-fitness score in Table 7.13. Then transfer that percentile score to the Summary Score Sheet.

was greater than the 60th percentile, color the corresponding thermometers *green*; for profiles in which your score was below 60th percentile, color the corresponding thermometers *red*. This way you can quickly obtain an overview of your profile ratings, both numerically and visually.

Next, in the lower half of the summary score sheet calculate your overall fitness rating. You do this by multiplying each of your profile ratings (copy them from the upper half of the score sheet) by a given profile-weighting component. Note that not all the profile areas are weighted equally. For example, aerobic fitness is regarded as the most important aspect of personal fitness and

SUMMARY SCORE SHEET:
PERSONAL FITNESS RATING

NAME _____ SEX _____ DATE _____

AGE _____ HEIGHT _____ MASS _____

SUMMARY OF INDIVIDUAL PROFILE RATINGS

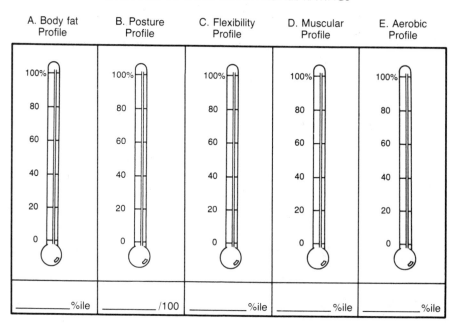

A. Body fat Profile	B. Posture Profile	C. Flexibility Profile	D. Muscular Profile	E. Aerobic Profile
_____%ile	_____/100	_____%ile	_____%ile	_____%ile

Composite Fitness Rating

PROFILES RANKED IN IMPORTANCE	profile rating		profile weighting		weighted rating
1. aerobic profile	_____	×	.30	=	_____
2. body-fat profile	_____	×	.25	=	_____
3. body dynamics: posture profile	_____	×	.15 ⎤		
flexibility profile	_____	×	.15 ⎦	=	_____
4. muscular profile	_____	×	.15	=	_____

Personal Fitness Rating: ⬚ _____/100

thus is given the greatest weighting (.30). Body fat is considered the second most important profile and is weighted accordingly .25. The remaining three profiles are weighted equally, at .15. Multiply each profile rating by its weighting component, and then place these weighted ratings in the space provided in the right-hand column. Total these weighted ratings; this sum is your overall fitness rating on a scale of 1 to 100 (a rating of 50 is considered average).

Suggested Stages for Evaluating your Personal Fitness

There are a number of methods for evaluating personal fitness, and we offer the following four stages as guidelines. Our overriding objective in doing so is to help you first to understand your fitness ratings and then to develop an appropriate exercise prescription in Chapter 8. At the completion of any of the stages you need not proceed to the next stage if you are satisfied with your evaluation and understanding of your ratings at that point.

First Stage. Enter your overall fitness rating in Figure 7.28. If your composite score is greater than 80 out of 100, you have superior overall fitness. More important, the two most heavily weighted profiles (aerobic and body-fat) most likely were also rated quite high. If you have an area of concern (see the second and third stages), it is probably in one of the other three profiles. If your composite score is between 60 and 80, your overall fitness is above average, but there is room for improvement, probably in either or both of the two most heavily weighted profiles. Finally, if your composite score is less than 60, your fitness results require the more in-depth analysis and direction provided by the second and third stages in order for you to develop an appropriate prescription in Chapter 8.

Second Stage. If your fitness rating is less than 80, you should further examine the profile(s) in which you scored the lowest. Therefore in the second stage of Figure 7.28 rank each profile according to its percentile rating: place the lowest-rated profile at the top of the column; place the highest-rated profile at the bottom; then rank the remaining three profiles 2nd, 3rd, and 4th accordingly. This hierarchy will enable you to make two analyses. First, it highlights the profiles where fitness improvements need to be made. If your fitness rating is above average (between 60 and 80), two profiles of concern will probably be highlighted. On the other hand, if your fitness rating is less than 60, you probably need improvement in the majority of the profiles. If so, you will have to decide which profile area(s) to concentrate on when you develop your prescription. The third stage of this evaluation is designed to help you make this decision.

Third Stage. In the third stage of Figure 7.28 rank the profile areas as you did in the second stage. Note, however, that each profile's weighting factor is included in this analysis. For example, if you scored at the 75th percentile in both the aerobic and muscular profiles, you would proceed as follows:

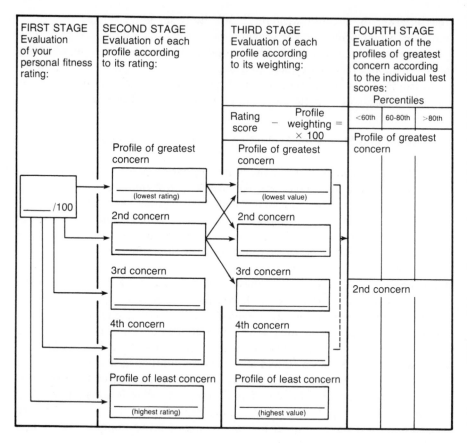

FIGURE 7.28 Evaluate your personal fitness rating sequentially according to the four stages indicated (see text for details). At the completion of any stage you need not proceed to the next.

aerobic fitness   = 75th percentile − (.30 × 100) = value of 45
muscular profile = 75th percentile − (.15 × 100) = value of 60

Therefore, you would place your aerobic-profile value above your muscular-profile value in the third-stage column. Stated another way, your aerobic fitness would be established as a greater concern than your muscular fitness. Thus the third stage offers three additional analyses:

1. The profile(s) requiring the greatest concern are highlighted.
2. A comparison of the second and third stages will enable you to highlight one or possibly two profiles (the one or two profiles ranked at or near the top in both stages) as the area(s) to improve *first* in your exercise prescription in Chapter 8.

3. Profiles whose third-stage values remain above 60 (as in the case of the muscular profile in the example above), need *not* be considered a concern. This touchstone is also the ultimate indicator of those persons who have achieved a very superior fitness rating: are all 5 of your values (i.e., every profile rating minus its weighting factor times 100) equal to or greater than 60? If so, you possess superior overall fitness and should develop a maintenance prescription from Chapter 8.

Fourth Stage. The final stage in this evaluation procedure involves an analysis of the individual test results that make up the profile ratings. For the profile(s) established as the greatest concern, find your percentile scores on the various tests from that profile and list them in the appropriate spaces in Figure 7.28. In this way you can determine specific deficiencies in various fitness areas, and this will help you develop a fitness prescription that is right for you from the activities, exercises, and prescription choices outlined in Chapter 8.

REFERENCES

1. American College of Sports Medicine, *Guidelines for Graded Exercise Testing and Exercise Prescription,* 2nd ed. (Philadelphia: Lea & Febiger, 1980), p. 1.
2. *Par–Q Validation Report* (Victoria: British Columbia Ministry of Health, 1978).
3. P.-O. Astrand and I. Rhyming, "A Nomogram for Calculation of Aerobic Capacity (Physical Fitness) From Pulse Rate During Submaximal Work," *Journal of Applied Physiology,* 7 (1954), 218–21.
4. B. Balke and R. W. Ware, "An Experimental Study of 'Physical Fitness' of Air Force Personnel," *United States Armed Forces Medical Journal,* 10 (1959), 675–88.

8

Personal
Fitness Prescription

INTRODUCTION

In this chapter we prescribe personalized fitness programs developed from scientific formula presented in this chapter. The total program you select should be suited to your fitness needs, as determined in Chapter 7. In personalizing your fitness program by means of the formula and instructions in this chapter, keep in mind a number of important principles. Most important, the intensity of any exercise must be suited to your present capacities. Exercise should never overstress; on the other hand, physiologically as you improve you will have to revise your prescription periodically. Second, from the exercise classifications in this chapter—warm-up and flexibility, calisthenics, strength, and aerobic—select exercises that are suited not only to your fitness needs but also to the type(s) of activity you desire. If, for example, you wish to forego jogging for more sports-oriented activity, you may turn to Chapter 9 for specific instructions on the amount and types of such activities. Finally, in order to gain optimal improvements from your program, remember to include in it the duration of each of the 4 phases and the appropriate number of repetitions of each exercise. If developed correctly, your program will accomplish two important objectives: it will introduce enjoyable activity into your lifestyle, and in 6 to 10 weeks it will bring about positive health and fitness results. The fundamental concepts and information upon which your program should be based are explained in Chapters 2–6.

GENERAL PRESCRIPTION FORMAT

Your prescribed program should be carried out 3 times per week or 5 times every 14 days. On alternate days, less strenuous activity is recommended: walking, cycling, swimming etc. Or perform only selected flexibility exercises that are outlined. The duration of the formal exercise sessions should be 30 minutes (minimum) to 60 minutes (maximum). More important, the time of day, location, and facilities must be suitable in terms of convenience, proximity, and time constraints. Thus during each 168-hour week, *only* 1.5 to 3.0 hours should be spent on formal exercise. This short period will prove to be one of your most healthful and enjoyable yet least expensive time investments.

Each formal exercise session should include the following phases: (A) *warm-up* (5–10 minutes); (B) *calisthenics* (5–10 minutes); (C) *aerobic exercise* (15–40 minutes); and (D) *cool-down* (5–10 minutes). The exact time of each phase will be determined by the specific exercises chosen and the prescribed times. You may also perform a phase E, *weight training,* at the end of phase B and/or the beginning of phase C, if you want to improve strength and muscular endurance in particularly weak areas of the body, as determined by your strength scores in Chapter 7. This general format is presented schematically in Figure 8.1.

A. Warm-up. The objective of this phase is to gradually increase total body movement in preparation for the more vigorous activity to follow. A proper warm-up will increase the temperature of the muscles and elevate the body metabolism, as well as help minimize possible injuries. Walking and slow running, followed by flexibility exercises, will achieve this objective. Several exercises are recommended; select only the ones best suited to your needs.

B. Calisthenics. The objectives of this phase are to enhance development in specific muscle groups and to increase muscular strength and endurance and the mobility of specific segments of the body. Many exercises are detailed; again, select only those that are specifically suited to your needs.

FIGURE 8.1 General format for exercise prescription. For specific reasons or on certain days you may wish to concentrate on a particular phase.

A. Warm-up	B. Calisthenics*	C. Aerobic exercise*	D. Cool-down
← 5–10 min. →	← 5–10 min. →	← 15–40 min. →	← 5–10 min. →	*total time = 30–60 min.*

*Weight training may be performed at the end of phase B and/or the beginning of phase C, up to 3 times per week

C. Aerobic Exercise. This phase should provide the main portion of the exercise prescription. Its objective is to elevate the functioning of the body's oxygen-transport system to an optimal level and to sustain this level for at least 15 minutes. A substantial number of calories are utilized thereby (10 to 15 percent of your daily caloric requirements is the recommended figure).

D. Cool-down. The sole objective of a cool-down exercise is to begin the body's gradual return to the resting state. As illustrated in Figure 5.6, the greatest physiological changes occur during the initial 5 to 10 minutes following exercise. Therefore, you should jog lightly or walk until your heart rate has returned to below 120 beats per minute. You may then perform limited flexibility exercises, particularly for the legs.

SPECIFIC EXERCISE PRESCRIPTION

Phase A. Warm-up

Definition. The first phase of an exercise session is the warm-up. This 5-to-10-minute session should activate the physiological systems in preparation for the more vigorous exercise to come.

Importance. There are a number of important reasons for including a warm-up in an exercise prescription. First, you should be mentally prepared for the exercises that are to follow, just as the elite athlete works hard, mentally as well as physically, prior to competition in order to perform his or her best. Further, increasing your body temperature by warming up reduces the incidence of injury to muscles and joints in subsequent strenuous exercise. The warm-up should also be designed so that it stretches out your muscles and allows your joints to move through their complete range of motion.

Prescription Principles. This phase of the exercise session should range from a light to a moderate level of intensity. The session should be divided into two parts: aerobic activities and stretching exercises.

1. The aerobic activities should be of low intensity, their speed and frequency dependent on your fitness level. The activities should be sufficient only to increase body temperature to the point where you feels warmer; any sweating at this point will be the result more of environmental conditions than of the activity itself (see Chapter 5).

2. The stretching exercises should be performed slowly and carefully. Select exercises that stretch all of the major joints and muscle groups of the body through their natural range of motion. Each exercise should be performed rhythmically (avoid bobbing and jerking) up to ten times. Or, if you prefer, hold the stretch position for 10 to 20 seconds, and repeat up to 5 times.

Prescription. The following aerobic and stretching exercises for the warm-up phase are only suggestions. The first is a normal warm-up for the less physically fit; the second is more suitable for active, physically fit people. The exercises may be replaced, modified, or expanded to include skipping, swimming, or some other activity, as long as the objectives for warm-up exercises are met.

Example of Aerobic Warm-up. The most common aerobic warm-up is a sequence of slow walking → walking → brisk walking → jogging → steady running → etc. However, a number of other innovative warm-ups can be developed, depending upon the facilities. In the house, for example, the following sequence is possible: walking up 1 to 5 flights of stairs (walk down) → slow running up stairs (walk down) → continuous two-leg jumping up stairs (walk down) → etc. Similar warm-up sequences can be devised for mediums such as water and snow.

Specific Flexibility Exercises. *Do not* overstretch—these are warm-up exercises.

For the Neck:

Exercise 1: Neck Rotator. Keeping the eyes focused forward and holding the chin in toward the neck, move the head slowly in a circular pattern, first in one direction and then in the other (Figure 8.2a). (Stretches neck rotators—flexors and extensors.) *Note*: If you have neck problems, avoid these exercises unless you are directed to perform them by a physician.

Exercise 2: Neck Twists. Turn the face slowly to the left and then to the right; repeat several times (Figure 8.2b). Stretches neck rotators—flexors and extensors.)

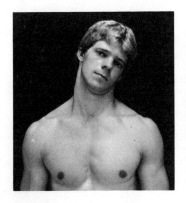 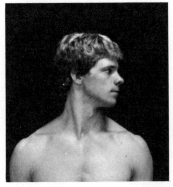

FIGURE 8.2
(a) Neck rotator.

FIGURE 8.2
(b) Neck twists.

For the Trunk:

Exercise 1: Twister.   Standing with feet apart and arms abducted sideways, twist to the left with arms and face moving in the same direction (Figure 8.3), and then twist to the right. Repeat slowly and rhythmically 5 to 20 times. (Stretches neck and trunk rotators.)

Exercise 2: Side Bender.   Standing with feet apart and hands on head, bend slowly from side to side in the frontal plane (Figure 8.4). Repeat 5 to 10 times. (Stretches lateral benders of trunk.)

Exercise 3: Front Bends.   Standing with feet together (Figure 8.5a), fully flex the neck, trunk, and hips and slightly flex the knees (Figure 8.5b). Extend, and repeat 5 to 10 times. (Stretches trunk, neck, and hip extensors.)

For the Legs:

Exercise 1: Hamstring Stretcher.   Sitting on the floor with legs straight and spaced, reach for one ankle and hold; do the same with the other ankle (Figure 8.6). Repeat 5 to 10 times. (Stretches hip extensors and knee flexors.)

Exercise 2: Lateral Stretcher.   Standing with legs wide apart and hands on hips, bend left leg and move body weight to the left; hold, and then shift weight over to the other foot (right knee bent) (Figure 8.7). Repeat 5 to 10 times. (Stretches hip adductors.)

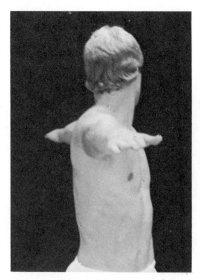

FIGURE 8.3 Twister.

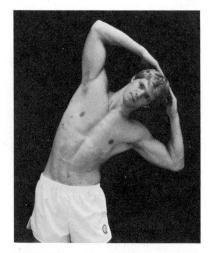

FIGURE 8.4 Side bender.

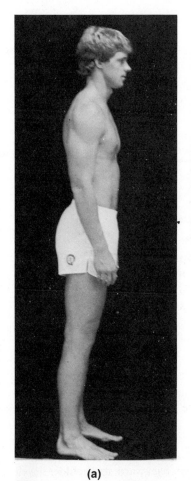

(a)

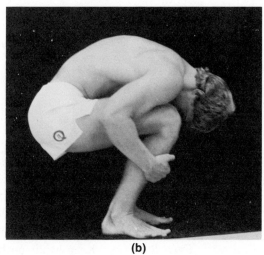

(b)

FIGURE 8.5 Front bends.

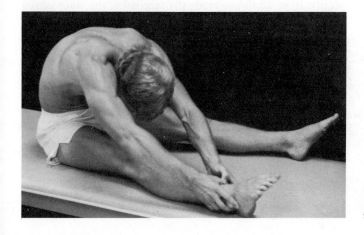

FIGURE 8.6
Hamstring
stretcher.

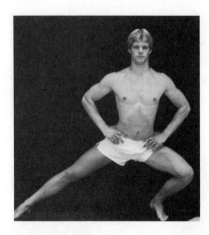

FIGURE 8.7
Lateral stretcher.

Exercise 3: Front Stretcher.   Keep hands on hips. Placing one leg (knee bent) well forward of the other (Figure 8.8) and keeping the other leg straight with ankle dorsiflexed, slowly move forward and hold for several seconds. Repeat 5 to 10 times for both sides. (Stretches the hip flexors, knee extensors, and ankle dorsi flexors.)

For the Shoulders:

Exercise 1: Arm Circles.   Standing with feet apart, perform slow, full-arm circles backward 5 to 10 times, then forward the same number of times. The arms should brush past the ears and the sides of the trunk (Figure 8.9). (Stretches the muscles crossing the shoulder joints.)

Exercise 2: Pull-Throughs.   Standing with feet apart, flex one arm (straight) forward to shoulder level, extend the other arm backward to shoulder level, then swing both arms down and through so that they reverse positions (Figure 8.10). Repeat rhythmically 10 to 20 times, gradually increasing the vigor of the

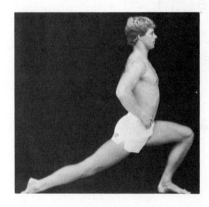

FIGURE 8.8
Front stretcher.

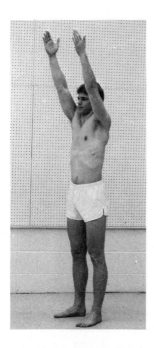

FIGURE 8.9
Arm circles.

pull-through and the flexion and extension of the shoulders. (Stretches the muscles crossing the shoulder joints.)

Phase B. Calisthenics

Definition. We define calisthenics as exercises that enhance development in specific muscle groups, increase muscular strength and endurance, and maintain or improve the mobility of specific segments of the body. You do not need apparatus in order to perform these exercises.

Importance. Calisthenics that are carefully selected can be useful in the development of muscular strength and endurance and joint mobility. Each exercise must have a purpose and benefit the individual who is performing it.

Prescription Principles. A calisthenic program should contain exercises that provide an overall development of the muscle groups of the body, as well as specific muscles where necessary. The session should systematically cover all the major muscle groups: the neck should be exercised through its full range of motion; the trunk, and thereby the trunk-flexor and trunk-extensor muscles, should be exercised in the sagittal plane; exercises should be provided for full range of motion for the spinal column in both the frontal and transverse planes; and exercises should be included for the legs and arms. Although the order in which you perform these calisthenics is not critical, performing them system-

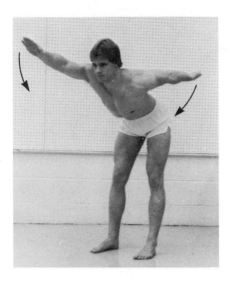

FIGURE 8.10
Pull-throughs.

atically helps ensure that all regions are worked and that no muscle group is overexercised at the expense of others. Table 8.1 summarizes the regions and muscle groups that are exercised.

The session should meet your needs and the exercises should not violate any principles of sound body mechanics (refer to Chapter 4). Specific exercises can be prescribed to correct functional postural defects and muscular imbalance and to help correct minor muscular weaknesses due to injury and other causes.

You can enhance the effects of the exercises by increasing the number of repetitions, the speed at which they are performed (most should not be performed quickly, however), and often by rearranging the mass or parts of the body in relation to the point of support (for example, doing a push-up in the more strenuous handstand position than in the regular position).

Cautions.   The human body is often able to tolerate tremendous impacts, such as automobile accidents, falls from great heights, and the repetitive clashes with other players in contact sports such as football, rugby, hockey, and boxing. On the other hand, you can become disabled by an injury caused by an impact or torque of comparatively little magnitude. You may sprain an ankle by overinversion, pull a hamstring muscle while jogging, or strain your back bending over to tie a shoelace, thereby putting the extensor muscles of the back into a painful and disabling spasm. Even exercises of mild to moderate intensity may result in pain and injury.

A number of calisthenics are not advisable for their intended purpose. Either avoid these exercises entirely, or perform them very carefully so as to reduce the potential for injury. The following are examples of such exercises.

Deep Knee Bend.   It has been claimed that the deep knee bend, or full squat, can injure the supporting structures of the knee, thereby often resulting in chronic

TABLE 8.1 Classification of Body Regions for Calisthenic Session

REGION	PLANE OF MOTION	MAJOR MUSCLE GROUPS
neck	sagittal	flexors
		extensors
trunk	sagittal	flexors
		extensors
	frontal	lateral benders
	transverse	rotators
legs	sagittal	flexors (hips)
		extensors (hips)
	frontal	abductors (hips)
		adductors (hips)
	sagittal	flexors (knees)
		extensors (knees)
		plantar flexors (ankles)
		dorsi flexors (ankles)
arms	sagittal	flexors (shoulders)
		extensors (shoulders)
	frontal	abductors (shoulders)
		adductors (shoulders)
	sagittal	flexors (elbow and wrist)
		extensors (elbow and wrist)

synovitis. The exercise unduly stresses the joints and ligaments of the knee, especially if it are performed vigorously.

If the objective of this exercise is to stabilize the knee joint by strengthening the knee extensors and flexors, then you can safely substitute half knee bends (knees and hips bend to 90 degrees), stair climbing, running, or hiking.

Supine Leg Raise.   This exercise is performed while lying on the back with the legs extended. The feet are raised about 30 centimeters (1 foot) off the floor and the position held. Variations of this exercise include opening and closing the legs, and flutter kicks that simulate the kicks used in swimming the back crawl. Leg raises have been used as abdominal strengtheners. However, during this exercise the weight of the legs is held predominately by the iliopsoas muscle, and unless the abdominal muscles are strong enough to maintain the position of the pelvis, keeping the lumbar vertebrae near the floor, the load will tilt the pelvis forward and hyperextend the lower back. Most young people possess a certain degree of lumbar lordosis that this exercise would accentuate. Older people, whose abdominal muscles may not be as strong as they should be, unduly stress the vertebrae of the lower back and may predispose themselves to disk herniation or other back injury by performing this exercise. Alternative exercise for strengthening the abdominal muscles are offered below.

Straight-Leg Sit-Up.   This exercise has an effect similar to that of the supine leg raise and should likewise be avoided.

Standing Toe Touch. This common exercise is often used *incorrectly* as an abdominal strengthener. Some people use it to stretch the trunk-extensor muscles in order to correct the lordotic curve in the lumbar region. The active muscle groups are the trunk and hip extensors: they contract concentrically and eccentrically throughout this exercise. The recoiling or bobbing at the fully flexed position excessively strains the hamstring muscles and their attachments as well as the muscles and ligaments supporting the lumbar vertebrae. If this exercise is to be done at all, bend the knees slightly; this will reduce the forces somewhat. Alternative exercises for stretching the trunk and hip flexors are provided below.

Prescription. We present two kinds of calisthenics: *general calisthenics* (exercises that improve or maintain joint flexibility and the endurance of the major muscle groups of the body) and *corrective calisthenics* (exercises that prevent or alleviate specific postural imbalances; these imbalances were discussed in Chapter 4 and evaluated in Chapter 7). Note that postural exercises are designed to strengthen the muscles involved in maintaining the desired posture and in stretching their antagonists. Perform these corrective exercises only after establishing that the deviation is *functional* rather than *structural* or pathological. Therefore, from the calisthenics outlined below, perform only specific exercises regularly, as needed.

1. General Calisthenics

These exercises are presented according to body region and muscle group (note Table 8.1).

For the Neck:

Exercise 1: Neck Flexor. Placing the fingertips on the forehead as in Figure 8.11a slowly flex the neck while applying resistance to the forehead. Repeat 2 to 10 times. (Exercises the neck flexors.)

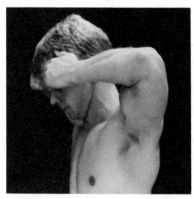
FIGURE 8.11 (a) Neck flexor.

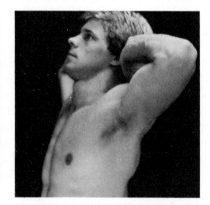
FIGURE 8.11 (b) Neck extensor.

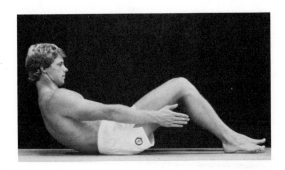

FIGURE 8.12
Trunk curls.

Exercise 2: Neck Extensor. Placing the cupped hands behind the head as in Figure 8.11b slowly extend the neck while tucking the chin in. Repeat 2 to 10 times. (Exercises the neck extensors.)

For the Trunk:

Exercise 3: Trunk Curls. Lying on the back with knees and hips flexed and arms extended at the side, flex the neck (leading with the head) and then the trunk to about 45 degrees, as in Figure 8.12; uncurl to about 20 degrees and curl again to 45 degrees. Repeat 5 to 30 times. A modification of this exercise is to place the hands on the head rather than having the arms extended at the side. This exercise should be done in lieu of the straight-leg sit-up exercise; it reduces the activity of the hip flexors (psoas muscles), which pull on the lumbar vertebrae, often causing discomfort to those predisposed to lower-back pain. (Exercises the trunk flexors.)

Exercise 4: Back Arches. Lying on the front with shoulders fully flexed (Figure 8.13), raise arms, head, and chest off floor and hold for 2 to 5 seconds. Repeat 5 to 20 times. Avoid this exercise if you have a lumbar lordosis. (Exercises the trunk extensors.)

Exercise 5: Side-Hand Lying. Balancing on hand of abducted arm and feet, lower and raise hips in frontal plane 5 to 20 times (Figure 8.14); change sides and continue. (Exercises lateral benders of trunk.)

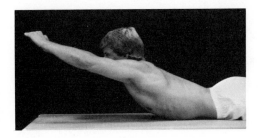

FIGURE 8.13
Back arches.

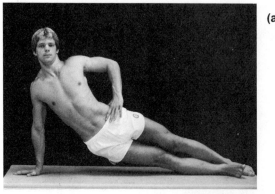

(b)

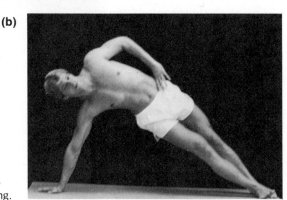

FIGURE 8.14
Side-hand lying.

Exercise 6: Stride Sitting, Trunk Twists. Sitting with legs extended and abducted and hands cupped behind head, rotate trunk from left to right, turning the head to look as far behind as possible on each turn (Figure 8.15). Repeat 5 to 20 times. (Exercises trunk rotators.)

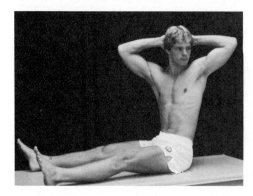

FIGURE 8.15
Stride sitting, trunk twists.

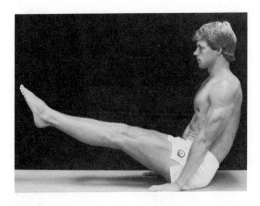

FIGURE 8.16
Leg lifts.

For the Legs:

Exercise 7: Leg Lifts. Sitting with legs extended and hands flat on floor next to hips (Figure 8.16), raise legs about 30 degrees off the floor and hold for 2 to 5 seconds. Repeat 5 to 20 times (Exercises hip flexors.)

Exercise 8: Hip Extensions. Kneeling with hands on floor, alternately extend legs backward and upward (Figure 8.17). Repeat 5 to 20 times. (Exercises hip extensors.)

Exercise 9: Stride Jumping. From a standing position, jump placing legs wide apart; jump again without pausing, bringing the legs back together (Figure 8.18). Repeat 10 to 20 times. (Exercises hip abductors and hip adductors.)

Exercise 10: Half-Squat Jumps. With hands on hips and knees bent to 90 degrees, jump straight up and land in starting position (Figure 8.19). Repeat with a 1-second delay 5 to 20 times. (Exercises knee extensors and knee flexors.)

Exercise 11: Ankle Rocking. In a standing position, raise the body as high as possible on tiptoes (Figure 8.20a), then lower; then lift toes and balls of feet off the floor, balancing on heels (Figure 8.20b); hold both positions for a few seconds. Repeat 5 to 20 times. (Exercises dorsi and plantar flexors of the ankles.)

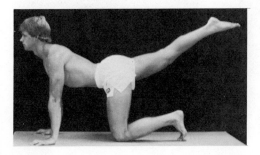

FIGURE 8.17
Hip extensions.

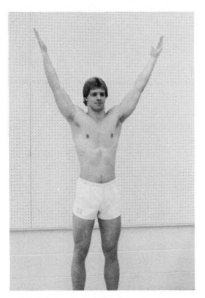

FIGURE 8.18   Stride jumping.

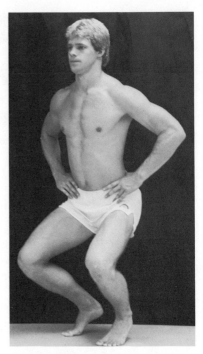

FIGURE 8.19   Half-squat jumps.

For the Arms:

Exercise 12: Push-Ups.   From a front lying position, elbows close to body (Figure 8.21a) perform slow push-ups with arms moving in sagittal plane (Figure 8.21b). Repeat 5 to 30 times. (Exercises shoulder flexors.)

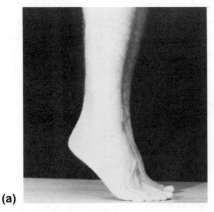

(a)

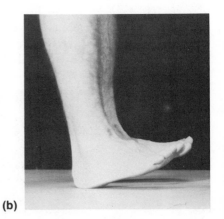

(b)

FIGURE 8.20   Ankle rockings.

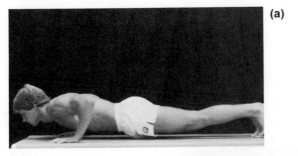

(a)

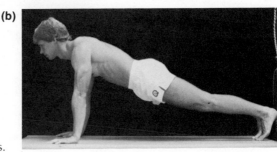

(b)

FIGURE 8.21 Push-ups.

Exercise 13: Hand Crawls. Kneeling with both hands on floor in front and head positioned between straight arms (Figure 8.22a), inch forward as far as possible by finger crawling (Figure 8.22b) and then work back to starting position. Repeat 5 to 10 times. (Exercises shoulder extensors.)

Exercise 14: Sideways Arm Swings. From a standing position, swing the arms sideways and up (Figure 8.23) and clap the hands above the head; then swing the arms back to the sides. Repeat 10 to 20 times. This can be done simultaneously with exercise 9. (Exercises shoulder abductors and shoulder adductors.)

Exercise 15: Clap Push-Ups. From a front lying position (Figure 8.24a), extend the elbows rapidly so that the body is lifted fairly high off the floor. Quickly clap the hands (Figure 8.24b) and replace them on the floor. Complete the push-up by returning to the starting position. Repeat 5 to 20 times. You can increase the difficulty by touching the hands to the chest instead of clapping them. (Exercises elbow flexors and elbow extensors.)

2. Corrective Calisthenics

The following exercises are provided in case you wish to plan an exercise prescription based on special needs arising from your posture profile in the last chapter. If your posture deviates significantly from the norm, consult your physician before performing the following corrective exercises.

Postural exercises are of little value unless the person doing them really

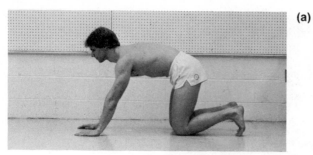

(a)

(b)

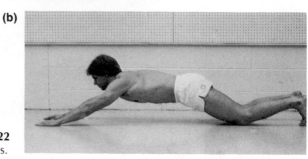

FIGURE 8.22
Hand crawls.

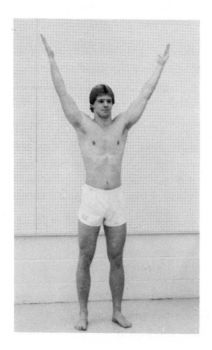

FIGURE 8.23
Sideways arm swings.

(a)

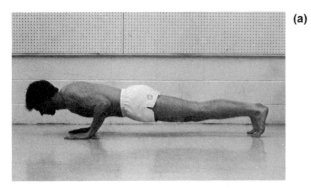

(b)

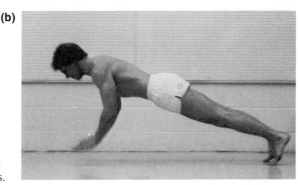

FIGURE 8.24
Clap push-ups.

wants to improve his or her posture: the exercises alone cannot remedy a condition caused by habitual poor body mechanics. One must continually be conscious of correct posture and attempt to improve his or her own posture.

Prevention and Correction of Forward Head:

Exercise 1: Neck Stretches.   Standing or sitting, flex the neck so that the chin is against the anterior aspect of the neck. Keeping the chin tucked inward, not downward, stretch the neck by attempting to raise the superior-posterior part of the head (Figure 8.25). Hold for a few seconds and then relax. Repeat 5 to 10 times. (Stretches neck extensors and strengthens neck flexors.)

Exercise 2: Neck Flattener.   Stand with the back leaning against a wall and the feet 30 to 50 centimeters in front. While pressing the back of the head against the wall try to flatten the neck. Keep the chin in and do not let the lower back leave the wall (Figure 8.26). Hold for a few seconds and then relax. Repeat 5 to 10 times. (Stretches neck extensors and strengthens neck flexors.)

Exercise 3: Neck Rotations.   Standing or sitting, rotate the head in a circle while holding the chin in (Figure 8.27). Avoid hyperextension of the neck. Rotate

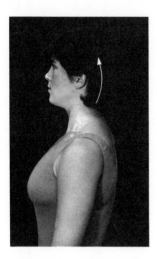

FIGURE 8.25
Neck stretches.

slowly 5 to 10 times in one direction and repeat in the other direction. (Exercises neck muscles.)

Exercise 4: Supine Neck Stretch.   Lying on the back with hips and knees well flexed and feet on floor, press head and neck against floor. (Figure 8.28). Keep the lower back flat on the floor. Hold the position for 5 seconds and then relax. Repeat 5 to 10 times. (Stretches neck extensors and strengthens neck flexors.)

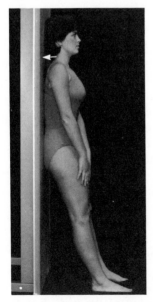

FIGURE 8.26
Neck flattener.

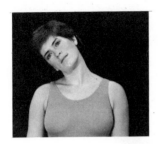

FIGURE 8.27
Neck rotations.

Prevention and Correction of Round Shoulders:

Exercise 1: Small Arm Circles. Standing with feet apart, arms abducted to the side, and forearms fully supinated (palms facing upward) (Figure 8.29) describe small circles backward, downward, forward, and upward. Attempt to stretch the pectoral muscles by keeping the circles as far backward as possible. Continue for about one minute and relax. Repeat 2 to 5 times. (Stretches pectoral muscles and increases flexibility of shoulder joints.)

Exercise 2: Large Arm Circles. Standing with feet apart, perform slow, full-arm backward circles. The arms should brush past the ears (Figure 8.30) and the sides of the trunk. Repeat 10 to 20 times. (Stretches the pectoral muscles.)

Exercise 3: Fall-Throughs. Standing 1 meter from a wall with feet apart, place hands on wall as in Figure 8.31. Slowly raise and lower the body, placing pressure on the shoulder extensors. Repeat 10 to 20 times. (Stretches the pectoral muscles).

Exercise 4: Hand Pulls. Standing or sitting with elbows raised to shoulder level, clasp hands and pull (Figure 8.32). Each arm resists the other in this isometric exercise. Hold tension for 5 to 10 seconds and relax. Repeat 5 to 10 times. (Strengthens horizontal abductors of shoulders and adductors of scapulae).

Exercise 5: Elbow Lifts. Lying prone, hands clasped behind head, raise head and shoulders off the ground; concentrate on lifting the elbows (Figure 8.33). Hold for 5 seconds and relax. Repeat 5 to 10 times. (Strengthens shoulder horizontal abductors and scapulae adductors and stretches pectoral muscles.)

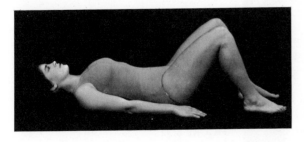

FIGURE 8.28
Supine neck stretch.

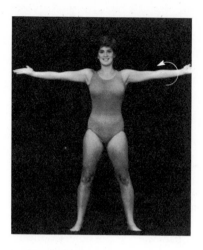

FIGURE 8.29
Small arm circles.

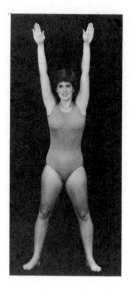

FIGURE 8.30
Large arm circles.

Exercise 6: Shoulder Flies. Lying prone on a narrow bench with arms hanging toward the floor, raise arms sideward and slightly forward as high as possible (Figure 8.34). Hold a few seconds and lower. Repeat 10 to 20 times. This exercise can be done holding a book, a brick or hand weights in each hand to increase the development of strength on the shoulder horizontal abductors and scapulae adductors).

Prevention and Correction of Lumbar Lordosis:

Exercise 1: Hip Stretches. Stand with one leg (knee and hip flexed) well forward of the other leg, which is extended as in Figure 8.35. With the trunk erect and the abdominal muscles taut, bob up and down gently and slowly for a minute. You should be able to feel some stretching anterior to the hip region of the

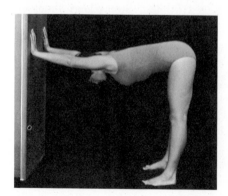

FIGURE 8.31
Fall-throughs.

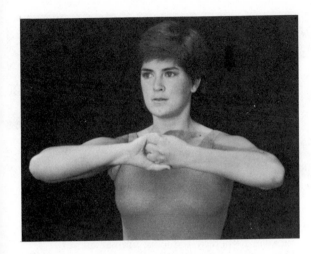

FIGURE 8.32
Hand pulls.

extended leg. Do the same with the other leg forward. Repeat 2 to 5 times for each leg. (Stretches the hip flexors.)

Exercise 2: Lumbar Stretch. Lying supine, flex both knees and hips to attain the starting position shown in Figure 8.36. Holding the legs straight, rhythmically extend and flex the hips through a range of 10 to 20 degrees. (Stretches trunk extensors in lumbar region).

Exercise 3: Lumbar Flattener. Lying supine with knees and hips slightly flexed, press lower back to floor by contracting abdominal muscles; keep neck and head in contact with floor. Hold for 5 to 10 seconds. Repeat 5 to 10 times. (Stretches trunk extensors and strengthens abdominal muscles.)

Exercise 4: Pelvic Tilt. While standing, contract the major hip extensors (glutei maximi) statically as hard as possible for approximately 5 seconds (Figure 8.37).

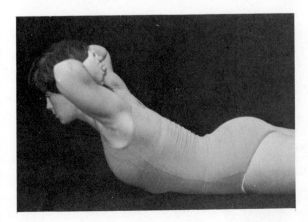

FIGURE 8.33
Elbow lifts.

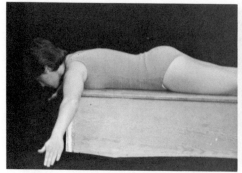 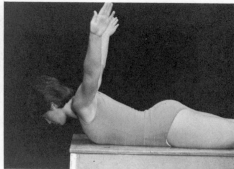

FIGURE 8.34   Shoulder flies.

Repeat 5 to 10 times. You may perform this exercise many times a day. (Strengthens hip extensors; tilts pelvis backward, thereby reducing lumbar curve).

Exercise 5: Mad Cat.   Kneeling with both hands on the floor (Figure 8.38a), contract the abdominal muscles so as to flatten the lumbar curve or even arch the spine upward like a mad cat (Figure 8.38b). Hold the position for 5 seconds. When returning to starting position avoid sagging the trunk. Keep the abdominal muscles fairly taut while resting. Repeat 5 to 10 times. (Strengthens trunk flexors and stretches trunk extensors in lumbar region.)

Exercise 6: Curl-Ups.   Lying supine with hips and knees flexed and arms at the sides a few centimeters off the floor, slowly flex the spine, starting with the neck, continuing with the upper back, and concluding with the lower back. The trunk should curl up so that the back is approximately 45 degrees to the floor (Figure 8.39). Repeat slowly 5 to 20 times. (Strengthens trunk flexors.)

   Variations:
a. Fold arms across chest.
b. Clasp arms behind head.

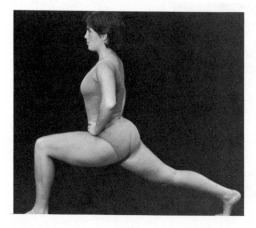

FIGURE 8.35
Hip stretches.

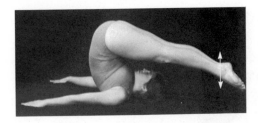

FIGURE 8.36
Lumbar stretch.

c. Clasp arms behind head; curl up with trunk twist so that left elbow touches right knee. Repeat, right elbow touching left knee, and continue to alternate.

d. Lying on floor with lower legs resting on the seat of a chair, flex knees and hips to 90 degrees; curl up as in original exercise.

Exercise 7: Hip Lift. Lying supine with hands clasping firm object and weight of legs directly over hip joints, lift the hips and lower back off the floor (Figure 8.40). Hold the position for 5 to 10 seconds. Repeat. (This is a very strenuous abdominal exercise and should be used only by those who have strong trunk flexors.)

Phase C. Aerobic Exercise

Definitions. It is universally agreed that maximal oxygen consumption is the best functional measurement of the health and fitness of one's oxygen-transport system. Since *aerobic* means "with oxygen," *aerobic exercise* implies activities

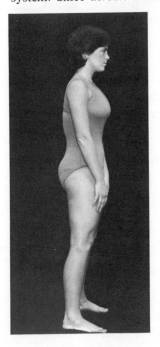

FIGURE 8.37
Pelvic tilt.

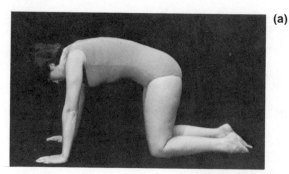

(a)

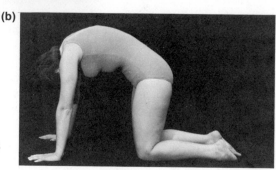

(b)

FIGURE 8.38
Mad cat.

that require oxygen transport and thereby improve the functional capacities of this system. Aerobic exercise must be of optimal intensity—that is, performed below one's anaerobic threshold and maintained for a specific period. This definition eliminates activities that are performed above an individual's anaerobic threshold or that are too mild.

Importance.   The physiological importance of correctly prescribed aerobic exercise is twofold: it places a healthful overload on the oxygen-transport system, and it expends from 10 to 15 percent of one's daily caloric requirements. In the following pages we outline criteria by which healthy adults can develop their own aerobic-exercise prescription.

Prescription Principles.   You must follow three principles in order to improve the functional capacities of your oxygen-transport system through safe and healthful aerobic exercise:

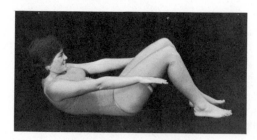

FIGURE 8.39
Curl-ups.

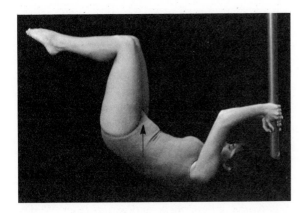

FIGURE 8.40
Hip lift.

1. The *intensity* (speed or rate) of the exercise must stress the oxygen-transport system while requiring minimal anaerobic-energy supplementation. Thus the intensity must be just below your anaerobic threshold, and this can be monitored accurately by means of your heart rate. Moreover, the intensity of the exercise must elicit your target heart rate, as outlined in Figure 8.41. If the intensity seems either too high or too mild, stop and quickly monitor your heart rate for 15 seconds (then convert to one minute). The heart rate you

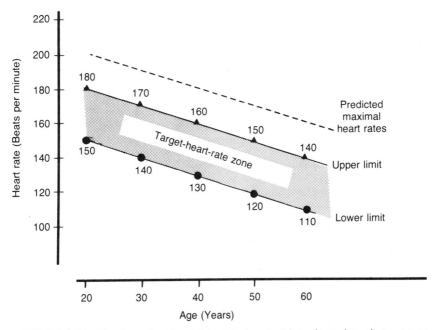

FIGURE 8.41 The intensity of aerobic exercise must be adjusted to elicit a target heart rate that falls between the upper and lower limits for one's age. *Source*: Fitness and Amateur Sport, Canada. Reprinted with permission.

recorded must fall within your target zone; if it does not, adjust the intensity of the exercise accordingly.

2. The *duration* of the exercise must be more than 15 minutes; that is, the exercise intensity (as defined above) must be sustained a minimum of 15 minutes. In most prescriptions the duration will usually be longer. The maximum duration of aerobic exercise cannot be defined as precisely; we recommend 40 minutes.

3. The *frequency* of the exercise should be 3 sessions every 7 days. Two modifications are possible: (a) 5 sessions spread out over 2 weeks; (b) 1 session every other day.

The options built into each of these principles accommodate these various phases of exercise prescription: *initiation, improvement,* and *maintenance.* Winter is a less active season for many; for others, office work can pile up at different times throughout the year. Whatever the reason, these persons may have to enter a maintenance phase in their exercise program: normal intensity (heart rate in the middle of their target zone), duration prolonged (30 to 40 minutes), but frequency reduced (5 aerobic sessions every 14 days). On the other hand, in spring and summer fitness enthusiasts usually prefer to embark upon an improvement phase: higher intensity (heart rate at the upper limits of their target zone), duration again prolonged, and frequency as high as 7 aerobic sessions every 14 days. At the other extreme, those beginning prescribed exercise start with an initiation phase: reduced intensity (heart rate elevated only to the lower limit of one's target zone—for persons who have been evaluated as unfit, this may necessitate only walking accompanied usually by weight reduction), reduced duration (15 to 25 minutes), and a frequency of either 3 sessions per week or 5 every 14 days. The initiation phase can be as long as the individual feels is necessary, or terminated when fitness reevaluation (Chapter 7) indicates that significant improvements have been made.

Prescription. By employing the calculations in the following chart* you can develop your own aerobic prescription. You need two pieces of data: your maximal oxygen consumption (see Chapter 7, score sheet E. 4) and your average daily caloric expenditure (see pp. 86–87). This prescription has direct application to running, specifying the distance to be run and the time in minutes in which that distance must be completed. However, if you do not wish to employ running, or if you prefer to vary the activities in the aerobic portion of your exercise prescription, you can apply the prescription developed below to other activities. Calculations are included in Chapter 9 for this purpose.

1. PERSONAL DATA:

Daily caloric expenditure = _____ calories

Maximal O_2 consumption = _____ ml O_2/kg./min.

* Adapted from D. A. Cunningham and P. A. Rechnitzer, *CAHPER,* 41 (1975), 25–31. Reprinted with permission.

2. DETERMINATION OF RUNNING DISTANCE:

This determination is based upon the amount of energy (in calories) you wish to expend during a session of aerobic exercise. First, select your target energy expenditure as a percentage of your daily expenditure. Use the following guidelines:

Phase of Exercise Prescription	Target Energy Expenditure: Percentage of Your Daily Energy Expenditure
initiation	11%
maintenance	13%
improvement	15%

Now determine your target energy expenditure in calories

$$\text{Daily caloric expenditure} \times \frac{\text{(target \% expenditure)}}{100} = \underline{\hspace{2in}} \text{ calories}$$

Finally, calculate the distance you must walk, jog, or run in order to expend this target energy:

$$\text{Distance} = \frac{\text{target energy expenditure (calories)}}{\text{body mass (kg.)}} = \underline{\hspace{2in}} \text{ kilometers}$$

Note: To convert this value to miles, divide by 1.61.

3. DETERMINATION OF RUNNING TIME:

Your speed is a function of your present maximal oxygen consumption. In Table 8.2, locate your maximum oxygen consumption in the left-hand column; then determine your running speed in the corresponding right hand column.

$$\text{Therefore the running time} = \frac{\text{Distance (km)}}{\text{Speed (km./hr.)}} \times 60 = \underline{\hspace{1.5in}} \text{ minutes}$$

4. SUMMARY OF PERSONALIZED AEROBIC PRESCRIPTION:

a. Distance (to be covered) is _____:___ kilometers.

b. Time is _____:___ minutes.

c. Speed is _____:___ km./hr. (from Table 8.2).

Phase D. Cool-Down

The purpose of the cool-down immediately following aerobic exercise is to help the heart rate gradually decrease to below 120 beats per minute. This will require 5 to 10 minutes. Therefore aerobic exercise should never end abruptly. Instead, after its completion there should be a gradual reduction in the intensity of activity. For example, if you were running, begin to jog, then walk rapidly, and then after 5 minutes begin moderate walking; discontinue this cool-down when your heart rate has slowed to below 120 beats per minute.

At this point you have a further cool-down option: perform a limited (3

TABLE 8.2   Walk/Jog/Run: Recommended Speeds for Both Males
and Females Based Upon their Maximal O_2
Consumption

MAXIMAL O_2 CONSUMPTION (ml./kg./min.)	PREDICTED SPEED (km./hr.)*	CATEGORY OF SPEED
20	5.0	
22	5.3	moderate to fast
24	5.7	walking**
26	6.1	
28	6.5	
30	6.9	
32	7.1	very fast walking***
34	7.3	
36	7.5	
38	7.7	
40	7.9	slow jogging
42	8.3	
44	8.7	
46	9.1	
48	9.7	normal jogging
50	10.3	
52	10.9	
54	11.5	
56	12.1	running
58	12.7	
60	13.4	

Source: Adapted from D. A. Cunningham and P. A. Rechnitzer, *CAHPER* 41 (1975), 25–31. Reprinted with permission.

*To convert value to miles per hour, divide by 1.61.

**If you were evaluated in Chapter 7 as having 25% body fat or curvature of the lower spine due to a protruding abdomen, you should use only walking speeds until you have reduced your body mass. Thus, select a slower speed to calculate your running time.

***If any of these speeds are uncomfortable, select a slightly faster or slower speed, whichever feels more comfortable. Use this speed in calculating your running time.

at most) number of specific flexibility exercises (see phase A of this chapter). These can serve two important purposes:

1. They can increase flexibility in areas of the body that you dare not exercise until you are fully warmed up (e.g., the hamstrings and the lower back).
2. They can gently restretch the muscles that have just performed the exercise. This technique has proved beneficial in helping specific muscles to "recover" after an exercise session.

Phase E. Strength Exercise

Definitions. Strength is defined as the maximum force that a muscle (or muscle group) can exert (see Chapter 3). Thus strength exercise is specific muscular activity designed to improve this capacity of the muscles. In this section, we further limit the definition, including only those muscular activities that require the use of implements (free weights, a Universal or Nautilus machine, etc.). (Exercises that use one's own body mass as the resistance appear in phase B of this chapter.)

Importance. Performing strength exercises has only *limited* importance, particularly in exercise prescription, since these exercises require minimal aerobic-energy expenditure. However, to a select number of persons strength exercise can prove beneficial:

1. most immediately, to individuals who perform either physically demanding work (lifting, loading, and so on) or who engage in recreational activities that demand strength (canoeing, backpacking, mountaineering, and so forth);
2. to persons who recorded major area(s) of weakness on their posture or muscular profiles (see Chapter 7) and who need to improve their strength in specific areas or muscle groups;
3. to males between 18 and 26, and to a growing number of females, who wish to improve the strength of major muscle groups.

Prescription. A specific muscle group must be isolated, as much as possible. (In practice, this is one of the advantages of strength machines versus free weights.) The muscles are then functionally overloaded by means of an implement, and repetitions of the exercise are performed. The load is repeatedly lifted against gravity through a predetermined range of motion (see illustrations in this section). Figure 8.42, illustrates the effects of functionally overloading a muscle group.

Strength improvements occur when only 1 to 5 repetitions of the load can be performed. On the other hand, more than 15 repetitions of a much lighter load will result in little strength improvement. Applying these principles of training, and for safety reasons, the resistance of the implement (free weights or machine) should be set so that a minimum of 5 but no more than 9 repetitions can be performed—this is called a *set.* To achieve the greatest improvement in the least number of sets, perform 3 sets of each strength exercise. The elapsed time between sets is relatively unimportant to the improvement of strength, and should be a matter of preference or governed by time restrictions.

To establish a functional overload for any strength exercise:

1. determine the present strength of the muscle group by performing one repetition of a maximal overload (but see the cautions outlined below).

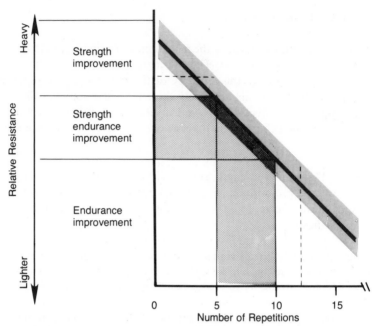

FIGURE 8.42   Relationship of strength improvements to the functional overloading of a muscle group: If a heavy resistance can be lifted only 3 to 5 repetitions (max.), muscular strength will improve. If a much lighter resistance can be lifted more than 10 to 12 times, muscular endurance will improve. Between these two extremes, specific to the load being lifted and the strength of the individual, both muscular strength and endurance improvements can result.

2. calculate 70 percent of that maximal overload; this will establish a load that can be lifted in 5 to 9 repetitions; this percentage will vary with the mass of the muscle group;

3. periodically redetermine your maximal overload (up to twice per month), and readjust the functional overload accordingly.

Prescription Summary:

One Set equals 5 to 9 repetitions of a specific strength exercise; this is the functional overload that improves strength.

Functional overload equals approximately 70 percent of one maximal overload; this percentage will vary with the mass of the muscle group.

Perform 3 sets to gain optimal strength improvements.

A maximum of 3 strength-exercise sessions should be performed over a 7-day period, on alternate days.

Cautions.   There are specific elements of risk in strength exercise. Exercises must be performed with correct technique; use the illustrations of the techniques as guides. Safety should always be a prime concern; use of strength machines or hand weights can greatly reduce the chance of accidents. Here are some specific safety measures:

1. Do not engage in strength exercise until you are fully warmed up—see phases A and B of this chapter. In this prescription, strength exercise should be performed only at the conclusion of phase B, as an adjunct to calisthenics, or in phase C, on the alternate days if strength exercises are to provide the major portion of the prescription.
2. Before performing exercises that require loads to be lifted overhead (military press, bench press, pull-overs, and so forth), make sure all equipment is operational and all adjustable pieces of equipment (free weights, weight collars, and so on) securely fastened.
3. When lifting a load greater than you own body mass, have an experienced spotter present (another person who can assist you). This is particularly important when determining your *maximal overload*, the heaviest load you can lift in a specific strength exercise.
4. Strength exercise should be carried out 3 times per week *at most*. Your muscles and body require at least 48 hours between sessions to recover fully. One or two sessions per week will provide adequate maintenance of strength.
5. Do *not* regularly attempt all the strength exercises illustrated below; select only the ones that suit your needs.

Exercises. These exercises are classifed according to regions of the body (see Table 8.3). Selection of particular strength exercises should be made accordingly. These regions are as follows:

1. Neck Region
2. Upper body—arms, shoulders, and chest musculature:
   a. Free-weight barbell exercises.
   b. Hand-weight exercises.

TABLE 8.3 Summary of Specific Strength Exercises According to Regions of the Body

EXERCISE	MAJOR MUSCLE GROUPS STRENGTHENED	MAIN MUSCLES EXERCISED	ILLUSTRATION IN THE TEXT
NECK REGION			
Neck Tuck	Neck Flexors	Sternocleidomastoid	Fig. 8.43
Neck Raise	Neck Extensors	Longissimus capitis	Fig. 8.44
		Semispinalis capitis	
		Splenius capitis	
UPPER BODY			
1. Free-Weight Barbell Exercises			
Biceps Curl	Elbow Flexors	Biceps brachii	Fig. 8.45
		Brachialis	
		Brachioradialis	*(Continued)*

TABLE 8.3 Summary of Specific Strength Exercises According to Regions of the Body (continued)

EXERCISE	MAJOR MUSCLE GROUPS STRENGTHENED	MAIN MUSCLES EXERCISED	ILLUSTRATION IN THE TEXT
	Wrist Flexors	Flexor carpi radialis	
		Flexor carpi ulnaris	
Triceps Curl	Elbow Extensors	Triceps brachii	Fig. 8.46
	Shoulder Extensors	Pectoralis major	
		Deltoid (anterior)	
		Latissimus dorsi	
	Wrist Flexors	Flexor carpi radialis	
		Flexor carpi ulnaris	
Bench Press	Elbow Extensors	Triceps brachii	Fig. 8.47
	Shoulder Horizontal Adductors	Pectoralis major	
		Deltoid (anterior)	
Military Press	Elbow Extensors	Triceps brachii	Fig. 8.48
	Shoulder Abductors	Deltoid (medial)	
Bent-Arm Pull-overs	Shoulder Extensors	Pectoralis major	Fig. 8.49
		Deltoid (anterior)	
	Elbow Extensors	Triceps brachii	
	Wrist Flexors	Flexor carpi radialis	
		Flexor carpi ulnaris	
Pull-Downs	Shoulder Adductors	Latissimus dorsi	Fig. 8.50
		Pectoralis major (sternal)	
	Elbow Flexors	Biceps brachii	
		Brachialis	
		Brachioradialis	
Upright Rowing	Shoulder Flexors	Coracobrachialis	Fig. 8.51
		Deltoid	
		Pectoralis (clavicular)	
	Elbow Flexors	Biceps brachii	
		Brachialis	
		Brachioradialis	
	Wrist Extensors	Extensor carpi radialis longus	
		Extensor carpi radialis brevis	
		Extensor carpi ulnaris	
Shoulder Shrugs	Shoulder-Girdle Elevators	Levator scapulae	Fig. 8.52
		Trapezius (upper)	
2. Hand-Weight Exercises			
Biceps Curls	Elbow Flexors	Biceps brachii	Fig. 8.53
		Brachialis	
		Brachioradialis	
	Wrist Flexors	Flexor carpi radialis	
		Flexor carpi ulnaris	
Triceps Curls	Elbow Extensors	Triceps brachii	Fig. 8.54
Bench Press	Shoulder Horizontal Adductors	Pectoralis major	
		Deltoid (medial)	
	Elbow Extensors	Triceps brachii	Fig. 8.55
Military Press	Shoulder Abductors	Deltoid (medial)	Fig. 8.56
	Elbow Extensors	Triceps brachii	

Shoulder-Fly
Exercise

Shoulder Flexors	Coracobrachialis	Fig. 8.57
	Deltoid	
Shoulder Abductors	Pectoralis (clavicular)	
	Deltoid (medial)	
Shoulder Horizontal	Pectoralis major	
Adductors	Deltoid (medial)	
Shoulder-Joint and	Deltoid (posterior)	
Shoulder-Girdle	Rhomboids	
Horizontal Abduc-	Trapezius	
tors		

TRUNK

Bent-Knee Sit-Ups	Trunk Flexors	Abdominals Iliopsoas Rectus femoris	Fig. 8.58
Good Mornings*	Trunk Extensors	Erector spinae Quadratus lumborum	Fig. 8.59

LOWER BODY

Half Squats	Knee Extensors Hip Extensors	Quadriceps Hamstrings Gluteus maximus	Fig. 8.60
Leg (Quadriceps) Extensions	Knee Extensors Hip Extensors	Quadriceps Hamstrings Gluteus maximus	Fig. 8.61
Leg (Hamstring) Curls	Knee Flexors	Hamstrings	Fig. 8.62
Heel Raises	Plantar Flexors	Gastrocnemius Soleus	

TOTAL BODY

Power Clean*	Plantar Flexors	Gastrocnemius Soleus	Fig. 8.63
	Knee and Hip Extensors	Quadriceps Hamstrings Gluteus maximus	
	Trunk Extensors	Erector spinae Quadratus lumborum	
	Elbow Flexors and Extensors	Biceps brachii Brachialis Brachioradialis Triceps brachii	
Dead Lift*	Shoulder Flexors	Coracobrachialis Deltoid Pectoralis (clavicular)	Fig. 8.64
	Shoulder-Girdle Elevators	Levator scapulae Trapezius (upper)	
	Wrist Flexors and Extensors	Flexor carpi radialis Flexor carpi ulnaris Extensor carpi radialis longus Extensor carpi radialis brevis Extensor carpi ulnaris	

*Avoid if you have back problems.

3. Trunk—abdominal and back musculature.
4. Lower body—buttock, thigh, hamstring, and calf musculature.
5. Total body: the exercises in this category require isotonic contractions by muscle groups from more than one region of the body. (In strength exercises, muscles in the other regions of the body must normally stabilize the joints, and therefore only contract isometrically.)

For the Neck Region:

Exercise 1: Neck Tuck.   Lying horizontally on the back, lift the free weight (wrapped in a towel) through a range of approximately 30 degrees (Figure 8.43).

Exercise 2: Neck Raise.   Lying prone (horizontal on the front), the Free Weight (wrapped in a towel) is lifted through a range of approximately 30 degrees (Figure 8.44).

For the Upper Body:

1. Free-Weight Barbell Exercises:

Exercise 1: Biceps Curl.   Standing with arms extended and grip supinated, lift barbell through 150 degrees (Figure 8.45). Do not allow the elbows to move, and minimize trunk movement.

Exercise 2: Triceps Curl.   Lying horizontal on the back and supporting barbell vertically overhead, grip pronated, lower barbell through a range of approximately 150 degrees about the elbow (Figure 8.46); then return barbell to the vertical. Minimize flexion of the shoulder.

Exercise 3: Bench Press.   Lying horizontal on back and supporting barbell vertically above, grip pronated, lower barbell to chest; then return (Figure 8.47). Minimize arching in the lower back.

Exercise 4: Military Press.   Standing with the barbell supported at shoulder height, grip pronated, lift barbell vertically over head to full extension of the elbows and shoulders (Figure 8.48); then return.

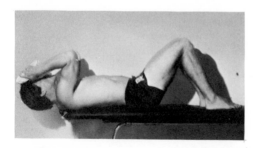

FIGURE 8.43
Neck tuck.

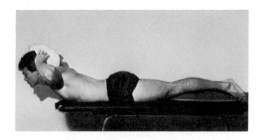

FIGURE 8.44
Neck raise.

Exercise 5: Bent-Arm Pullovers. Lying horizontal on back and supporting barbell across the chest, grip pronated, lift barbell over head and lower to full extension of the shoulder joints (Figure 8.49); then return. As much as possible, maintain at least a 90-degree (or less) angle in the elbow.

Exercise 6: Pull-Downs. Use a strength-exercise machine. Kneeling, taking a wide (pronated) grip on the bar, pull down until the bar touches the back of the shoulder, then return (Figure 8.50).

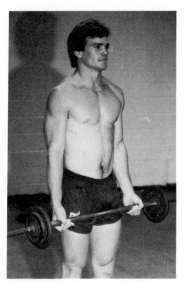

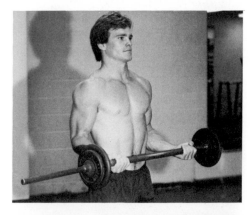

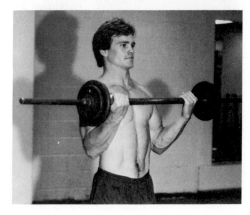

FIGURE 8.45
Biceps curl.

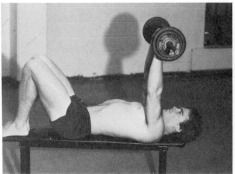
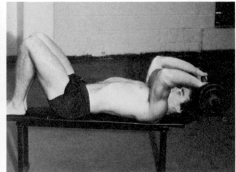
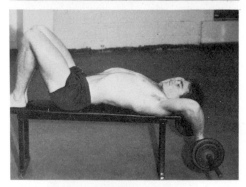
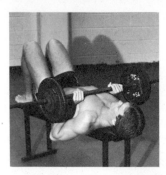

FIGURE 8.46
Triceps curl.

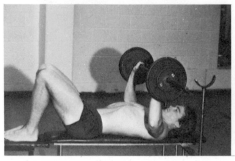

FIGURE 8.47
Bench press.

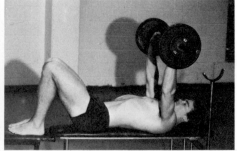

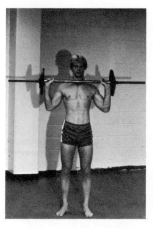
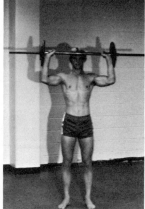
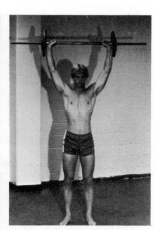

FIGURE 8.48 Military press.

Exercise 7: Upright Rowing. Standing with arms extended and grip pronated, lift barbell vertically as high as possible (Figure 8.51); then return.

Exercise 8: Shoulder Shrugs. Standing with arms extended and grip pronated, lift barbell only by elevating the shoulders (Figure 8.52). Keep the elbows locked.

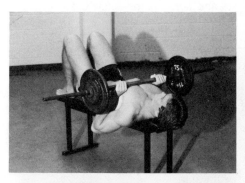
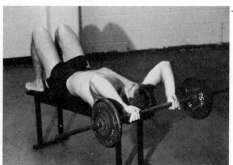
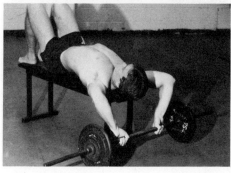

FIGURE 8.49
Bent-arm pullovers.

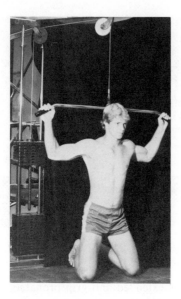

FIGURE 8.50
Pull-downs.

2. Hand-Weight Exercises: The first four barbell excerises for the upper body—
biceps curl, tricep curl, bench press, and military press—can be performed with
hand weights in place of barbells. For instructions on performance, see the
preceding descriptions of these exercises and note Figures 8.53–8.56.

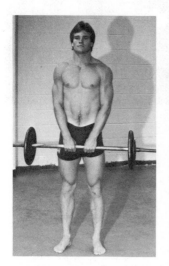 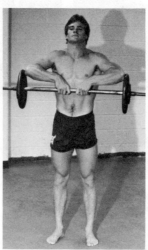 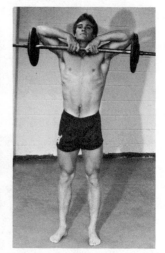

FIGURE 8.51   Upright rowing.

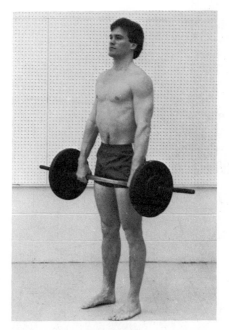 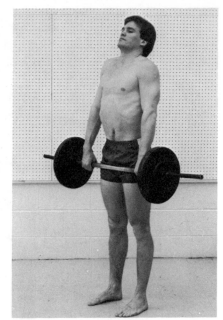

FIGURE 8.52 Shoulder shrugs.

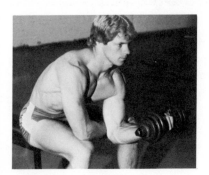

FIGURE 8.53
Biceps curls, with hand weights.

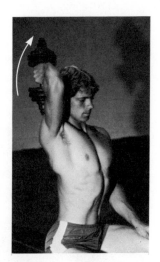

FIGURE 8.54
Triceps curls, with hand weights.

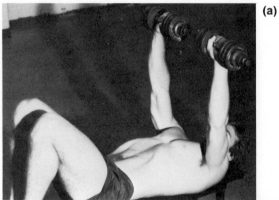

(a)

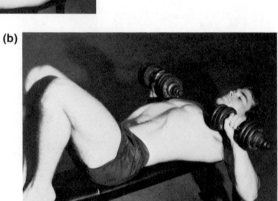

(b)

FIGURE 8.55
Bench press, with hand
weights.

Shoulder-Fly Exercise.   This is a series of separate exercises; select only the ones
best suited to your needs. (See Figures 8.57a–e).

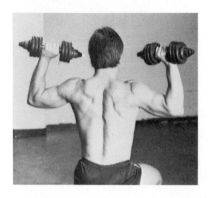

FIGURE 8.56
Military press, with hand
weights.

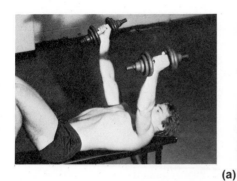
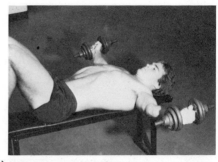

(a)

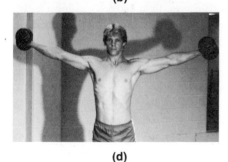

(b)

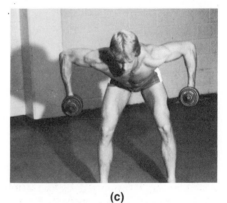

(c)

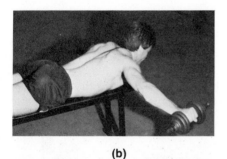

(d)

FIGURE 8.57 Shoulder-fly exercise: (a) lying supine, raise and lower hand weights sidewards; (b) lying prone, raise and lower hand weights sidewards; (c) standing bentover, arms hanging, lift hand weights vertically to shoulder level, then return; (d) standing, raise and lower hand weights sidewards; (e) standing, raise and lower hand weights frontwards.

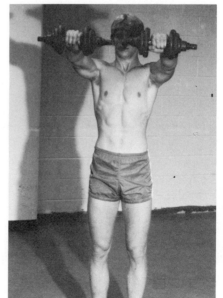

(e)

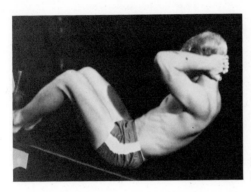

FIGURE 8.58
Bent-knee sit-ups.

For the Trunk:

Exercise 1: Bent-Knee Sit-Ups. Lying horizontal on back with free weight (wrapped in towel) behind head and toes firmly affixed under a foot support, sit up in a "rolling" fashion until elbows touch knees; then return (Figure 8.58).

Exercise 2: Good Mornings. Standing with a very light barbell resting on the shoulders and supported by the arms, grip pronated, bend forward until the hips are flexed at approximately 90 degrees (Figure 8.59). Keep the knees slightly bent, and do not overbend at the waist. Avoid this exercise if you have lower-back problems.

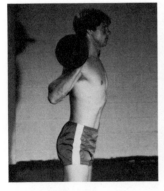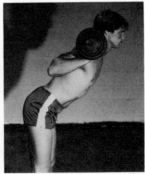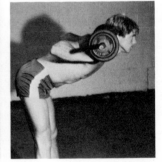

FIGURE 8.59 Good mornings.

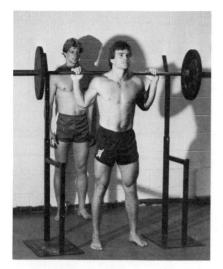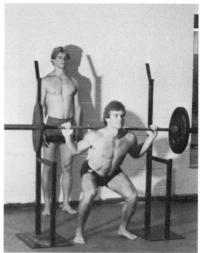

FIGURE 8.60   Half squats.

For the Lower Body:

Exercise 1: Half Squats.   Standing with heavy barbell resting on shoulders and supported by arms, grip pronated, bend at the knees to approximately 90 degrees, holding the back straight (Figure 8.60); then return.

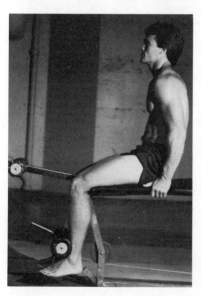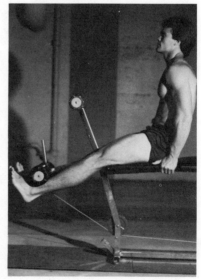

FIGURE 8.61 Leg (quadriceps) extensions.

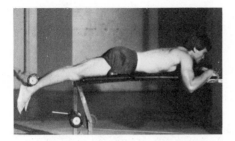

FIGURE 8.62 Leg (hamstring) curls.

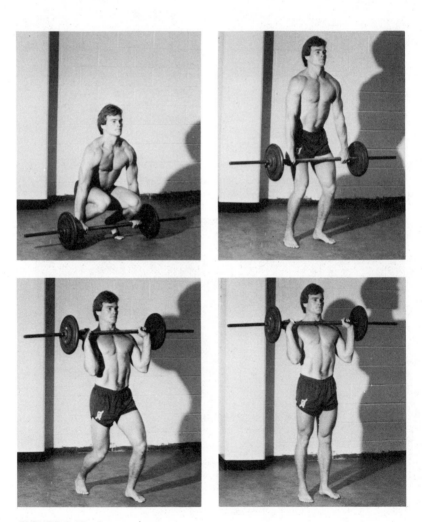

FIGURE 8.63 Power clean.

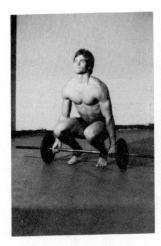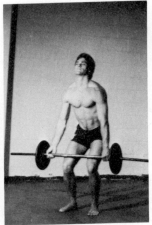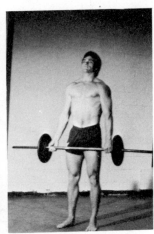

FIGURE 8.64 Dead lift.

Exercise 2: Leg (Quadriceps) Extensions. Sit on a strength-exercise machine, position adjusted so that the ankles are hooked in behind the padded supports. Holding firmly onto the seat, extend the knees until the legs are straight (Figure 8.61); then return.

Exercise 3: Leg (Hamstring) Curls. Lying supine on a strength machine, position adjusted so that the heels are hooked under the padded supports, flex the knees until the lower leg is vertical, 90 degrees at the knee (Figure 8.62); then return.

Exercises for Total Body Strength:

Exercise 1: Power Clean. With barbell resting on floor, bend at the knees and waist, grasp barbell with a pronated grip, and perform the sequences outlined in Figure 8.63.

Exercise 2: Dead Lift. With barbell resting on floor, bend at the knees and waist, grasp barbell with an interchanged grip (one hand pronated, the other supinated), and perform the sequence outlined in Figure 8.64.

9

Alternative Activity Prescriptions

INTRODUCTION

This chapter consists of alternative activity prescriptions for the aerobic phase of your exercise program. These alternatives are designed for persons who do not wish to follow the personalized running prescription developed in Chapter 8, and for others who are well along in their exercise prescription. For the latter group, advanced running prescriptions can be developed that employ either continuous running or higher-intensity interval running. The individualized prescriptions presented in this chapter are still based upon the personalized aerobic prescription developed in Chapter 8; only the activities are different.

ALTERNATIVE RECREATIONAL ACTIVITIES AND SPORTS

Table 9.1 lists several popular North American activities and sports. If you developed your own exercise prescription in Chapter 8, phase C, but do not wish to jog (or to jog exclusively at each exercise session), you may substitute one of these activities and use the following prescription formula:

Alternative Aerobic Prescription

1. Find the target caloric expenditure that you developed in Chapter 8, phase C. This provides the basis upon which the alternative activities are prescribed.

198

Target caloric expenditure = _____ calories

2. Select your preferred recreational activity or sport from Table 9.1.
3. Determine the amount of time for your participation per session:

$$\text{Time of participation (per session)} = \frac{\text{Target Energy Expenditure (calories)}}{\text{body mass (kg.)} \times \text{factor (from Table 9.1)}}$$

Therefore:

Participation time = _____ minutes ÷ 60 = _____ hours

This prescription is not meant to apply to competition at elite levels. However, if you maintain normal to vigorous intensity the activity or sport will provide an equivalent aerobic prescription.

ADVANCED RUNNING PRESCRIPTIONS

The remainder of this chapter consists of two advanced running prescriptions that you can substitute in phase C of your fitness prescription *twice* per week. They are intended for those persons who have been exercising regularly for at least 1 year and wish to (1) progress to a more advanced prescription or (2) initiate a *further* improvement phase. Persons who attempt either of these advanced prescriptions should have achieved superior scores (at least the 75th

TABLE 9.1 Popular North American Recreational Activities and Sports: Select Your Preferred Activity or Sport, and then Insert the Factor Opposite It Into the Formula for Alternative Aerobic Prescription

ACTIVITY/SPORT	FACTOR*	ACTIVITY/SPORT	FACTOR*
Backpacking	.045	Sailing	.021
Badminton	.037	Skating (recreational)	.038
Baseball	.035	Skiing: Cross-Country	.077
Basketball	.046	Downhill	.064
Bicycling	.071	Skipping	.061
Bowling	.044	Soccer	.057
Canoeing	.046	Swimming (length of pool,	.051
Disco Dancing	.039	front crawl)	
Golf (time for 18 holes)	.036	Tennis	.046
Handball	.064	Touch Football	.055
Hockey (playing time)	.068	Volleyball	.038
Racket Sports:		Water skiing	.051
Paddelball	.064	Wrestling	.085
Racquetball	.063		
Squash	.068		
Rock Climbing	.065		
Rowing	.035		
Rugby	.059		

*Mean caloric expenditure for these activities, in cal./kg./min.

percentile) on both their cardiovascular and body fat profiles in order to be sure they can perform it safely.

Your Aerobic Prescription: Summary

The prescription you developed in Chapter 8, phase C, is the basis for your advanced running prescription. Summarize the following data from your prescription:

Prescribed distance   =   _____   kilometers
Prescribed time   =   _____   minutes
Prescribed speed   =   _____   kilometers per hour

Advanced Prescription 1: High-Intensity Running— Continuous

This prescription employs continuous running at a faster speed and for a longer distance than those prescribed in Chapter 8. Take the aerobic prescription that you just summarized and modify it as follows:

Running distance:

total distance = _____ km. × 1.5
                    (prescribed distance)

             = _____ kilometers

Running intensity:

running speed = _____ km./hr. × 1.25
                    (prescribed speed)

             = _____ kilometers/per hour

Running time:

total time   = $\dfrac{\text{total distance (km.)}}{\text{running speed (km./hr.)}}$ × 60

             = _____ minutes

Frequency.   Advanced prescription 1 should be performed in conjunction with your regular aerobic prescription, according to the following schedule; the actual days of the week may be switched but the sequence should remain constant:

Monday	Tuesday	Wednesday	Thursday	Friday	Saturday	Sunday
Activity	Regular R$_x$	Activity	Advanced R$_x$ 1	Rest	Regular R$_x$	Advanced R$_x$ 1

←————————— work week —————————→ │← —— weekend ——— →│

Advanced Prescription 2: High-Intensity Running—Interval

This advanced prescription employs even more intense running (a faster speed) than advanced prescription 1. It is intended to elicit a physiological response above the anaerobic threshold. This prescription, therefore, *cannot* be carried on continuously; rather, *relief intervals* must be interspersed between the *run intervals*. (For an understanding of interval exercise, see Chapter 5.) Again, to develop advance prescription 2, modify your aerobic prescription from Chapter 8 using the calculations shown below:

Running distance:

total distance = _____ km. ÷ 0.5 = _____ kilometers
(prescribed distance)

Running intensity:

running speed = _____ km./hr. × 2.0 = _____ kilometers per hour
(prescribed speed)

Number of run intervals:

1. Length of each run interval:

   weeks 1 and 2 = 50 meters
   weeks 3 and 4 = 100 meters
   weeks 5 and 6 = 150 meters
   weeks 7 and 8 = 200 meters
   .
   .
   .
   .
   maximum distance = 400 meters

   Note: After week 4 it is up to you as to how much further you wish to keep increasing the run-interval distance.

2. Therefore, the number of run intervals = $\dfrac{\text{distance (kilometers)} \times 1000}{\text{length of 1 run interval (meters)}}$ =

   _____ number of intervals

Total time of exercise:

1. Time of 1 run interval =

$$\frac{\text{run-interval distance (meters)}}{\text{speed of running (km./hr.)}} \times 3.6 = \underline{\qquad} \text{ seconds*}$$

2. Time of 1 relief period =

time of 1 run interval (seconds) $\times 4^{**} = \underline{\qquad}$ seconds

3. Total run-interval time =

$$\frac{\begin{array}{c}\text{time of 1 run}\\\text{interval (seconds)}\end{array} \times \begin{array}{c}\text{no. of run}\\\text{intervals}\end{array}}{60 \text{ seconds}} = \underline{\qquad} \cdot \underline{\qquad} \text{ minutes}$$

4. Total relief-interval time =

$$\frac{\begin{array}{c}\text{time of 1 relief}\\\text{period (seconds)}\end{array} \times \begin{array}{c}\text{no. of run}\\\text{intervals}\end{array}}{60 \text{ seconds}} = \underline{\qquad} \cdot \underline{\qquad} \text{ minutes}$$

5. Approximate total time of exercise   = _____.____ minutes
                                                 (sum of steps
                                                 3 and 4)

*Calculate time to the nearest second.
**Employ a 1-to-4 run relief ratio; this may be decreased to 1-to-3.

Frequency.   Advanced prescription 2 should be performed in conjunction with regular aerobic prescription, according to the following schedule; the actual days of the week may be switched but the sequence should remain constant.

Monday	Tuesday	Wednesday	Thursday	Friday	Saturday	Sunday
Activity	Regular R_x	Activity	Advanced R_x 2	Rest	Regular R_x	Advanced R_x2

|← —————————— work week ——————————→ | ← —— weekend ——→ |

Glossary

abdominal muscles The trunk-flexor muscle group that forms the supporting wall for the organs of the abdomen and pelvic regions.

abduction Movement of a body segment in the frontal plane away from the midline of the body.

acromion Bony process on the superior/lateral aspect of the scapula (shoulder blade).

adenosine triphosphate (atp) The high-energy compound, found in all cells, that provides the most direct form of energy for the cell.

adipose tissue The body's fat-storage depots located subcutaneously (immediately under the skin) at certain areas, such as the buttocks and breasts.

adolescence Generally, the period from age 12 to age 18, commencing with puberty.

aerobic Means "with oxygen." Thus during aerobic exercise a large portion of the required energy is obtained from the aerobic-energy system (see oxygen-transport system). The aerobic capacity is the maximal amount of energy that can be produced by this system.

alveoli The 3 to 4 billion air sacs in the lungs where oxygen and carbon dioxide are exchanged between air and blood.

anaerobic Means "without oxygen." Thus in anaerobic exercise a large portion of the required energy is obtained from the anaerobic-energy sources. Anaerobic energy is required in high-intensity, short-term exercise involving power or speed (see *glycolysis anaerobic*).

anaerobic threshold That point where anaerobic energy begins to supplement the already sizable aerobic contributions.

anthropometry The study of human-body measurements, especially on a comparative basis, through determination of the dimensions of the body.

antigravity muscles The large extensor muscles that counter the tendency of the body to collapse due to the pull of gravity.

arteriosclerosis The advanced stage of atherosclerosis: main arteries harden and their internal diameter narrows.

artery A pressurized tube that transports blood away from the heart.

atherosclerosis The buildup of fat on the inner walls of the arteries.

atrium (pl. atria) One of the upper chambers of the heart. The right atrium receives venous blood from the systems of the body and the left atrium receives oxygenated blood from the lungs.

basal metabolic rate (bmr) The minimal amount of energy required to maintain the life processes of the body at rest; always determined in a fasting state.

blood pressure The force that the blood exerts against the walls of the blood vessels as it passes through them.

body composition The percentages of muscle, bone, fat, and other tissues that make up the body.

body density Body mass divided by body volume.

body fat See *fat*.

body mass The quantity of matter in a body; measured in kilograms.

body surface The total outer area (BSA) surface of the body, expressed in square meters (m^2).

body weight The gravitational force exerted on a body by the earth. Whereas the *mass* of a body does not change from one place on the earth to another, *weight* varies slightly from place to place. (If the mass of a person is 70 kilograms, then the weight of the person would be 70 kilograms $\times$ 9.81 meters/second = 686.7 newtons [N].)

bronchial tubes The two air tubes that branch off from the trachea to each lung.

calisthenics Exercises performed for the purpose of muscular development and/ or flexibility without the use of implements.

calorie A unit of energy; 1000 calories (kilocalorie [C]) is the usual unit of measure in discussions of body metabolism.

capillary Smallest division of the circulatory system; the tiny tubes where oxygen and nutrients are transferred from the blood to the cell and where the waste products of metabolism are transferred from the cell to the blood.

carbohyrate An energy food found in the body in the forms of glucose and glycogen obtained from sugars and starches.

carbon–dioxide production Results from aerobic metabolism; while oxygen is being utilized by the working muscles, a similar volume of carbon dioxide is being produced, transported (by the blood) to the lungs, and exhaled.

cardiac output The volume of blood pumped by the heart per minute; equals heart rate times stroke volume.

cardiorespiratory Referring to the heart and lungs.

childhood Generally, the period from age 4 to the onset of puberty (approximately age 12).

cholesterol A biochemical that is vital to normal body function. However, excess blood cholesterol has been associated with heart and vascular disease.

circuit training A sequence of exercises or activities performed at individual stations within a given time limit.

concentric contraction An isotonic contraction in which the muscle shortens while it produces tension.

conditioning Physical training; *not* synonomous with *exercise prescription.*

cool-down The last phase of an exercise prescription which helps the body to return to its normal metabolic state immediately after exercise.

coronary arteries The main arteries that supply the heart muscle with blood. Impairment or blockage of these arteries can lead to coronary heart disease.

dehydration Excessive loss of body fluids.

diastolic blood pressure The lowest pressure exerted by the blood against the walls of the arteries; usually measured on the upper arm just above the elbow, at the level of the heart.

diuretic A chemical that increases urine output in order to reduce the total amount of fluid in the body.

duration The length of time one should exercise; one of the key variables of exercise prescription.

eccentric contraction An isotonic contraction in which the muscle is lengthening while producing tension (for example, lowering a mass while resisting gravity).

electrocardiogram (EKG) A tracing (for permanent record) of the electrical activity of the heart, including heart rate.

endorphins A class of biochemicals released into the body from the pituitary and other tissues; they have an opiate-like effect.

endurance The ability to carry out moderate to heavy physical activity over an extended period; the primary energy source for endurance exercise is the aerobic system.

enzyme A biochemical, predominantly protein, that speeds up a chemical re-action of the body.

epicondyles Round articular processes on the ends of long bone at the joints.

ergometer An exercise devise (usually a stationary bicycle).

esophagus The flaccid tube through which food passes from the mouth to the stomach.

exercise prescription A 4-phase individualized exercise program; different from training and conditioning, which are sports-related concepts.

extension Movement of a body joint such that the angle about the center of rotation (the fulcrum) increases.

fast-twitch muscle fiber The type of muscle fiber used for sudden powerful bursts of activity.

fat Fatty acids are long-chain-carbon foods obtained from animals and con-sumed for energy production. *Body fat* consists of most of the unmetabolized energy foods (excess carbohydrates, animal fats, and protein) stored in the body in the form of *tryglycerides.*

fat-free mass See *lean body mass.*

fat mass The quantity of body fat, usually expressed as a percentage of total body mass.

flexibility The range of movement about a body joint.

flexion Movement of a body joint such that the angle about the center of rotation (the fulcrum) decreases.

frequency Number of exercise sessions per week; one of the key variables of exercise prescription.

glucose The six-carbon sugar found in the body.

glycogen The form in which glucose molecules are stored in the body; made up of thousands of glucose molecules attached one to the next—an economical way to store the body's limited supply of glucose, mainly in the liver and muscles.

glycolysis anaerobic The metabolic pathway in muscle that breaks down sugars (specifically glucose and glycogen) very rapidly into lactic acid, thereby liberating the large amounts of energy necessary for speed and power activities.

gram A basic unit of mass in the metric system. One thousand grams equal 1 kilogram.

heart rate The number of times per minute that the heart fills with blood and then pumps it into the vascular system.

hematocrit Blood is approximately 40 percent hematocrit. The solid (nonfluid) component of blood.

hemodynamics The movement of blood (a viscous liquid) through the vast tubular network of the body.

hemoglobin The element in the red blood cell that chemically combines with the oxygen in the lungs and then releases that oxygen to the tissues of the body.

high–density lipoprotein–cholesterol A form of cholesterol, found in the blood plasma, that is increased by regular exercise and that may protect against heart disease.

hormones Biochemicals produced by specialized cells and tissue in the body that are vitally important in controlling the metabolism of other cells and tissues.

hyperextension Movement of a body joint such that the angle about the center of rotation (the fulcrum) increases beyond 0 degrees.

hypertension An abnormally high blood pressure at rest (a systolic pressure > 140 mmHg and a diastolic pressure > 90 mmHg).

hypertrophy An increase in the size or mass of a cell, tissue, or organ.

iliac crest The large bony prominence at the top of each side of the hips.

intensity Degree of vigor of any phase of an exercise prescription—mild, moderate, maximal, and so forth; one of the key variables in exercise prescription.

intermittent exercise Activities performed with alternate periods of intense activity interspersed with short rest periods.

interval training Repeated bouts of exercise performed at an intensity above the anaerobic threshold, alternated with periods of rest or light exercise.

isometric contraction Contraction in which a muscle generates tension with no overt movement.

isotonic contraction Contraction in which a muscle generates tension while shortening or lengthening.

kgm./min. Kilograms times meters per minute. A kilogram-meter (kgm) is a measure of work (which is defined as moving a mass through a distance), and thus kilogram-meters per minute is the rate of doing work.

kilogram   Metric unit of mass; equals 1000 grams.

lactic acid   A product of anaerobic metabolism. It results from the rapid breakdown of sugars (specifically glycogen and glucose) in the muscles during intense exercise. As lactate builds up in the muscles it diffuses into the blood.

lean body mass   (also referred to as fat-free weight) That portion of the body mass that is not body fat (muscle, skeleton, and connective and organic tissues).

ligaments   The main connective tissue of the body that connects bones.

lipid   A category of body fat; includes fatty acids, triglycerides, and cholesterol.

lipoprotein   A protein that has combined chemically with cholesterol or triglycerides in the bloodstream.

liter   The unit of volume in the metric system.

lungs   The organ that accommodates the exchange of oxygen and carbon dioxide between the blood and the external environment.

maximal aerobic capacity   Maximal oxygen consumption (Vo_2 max); the maximal amount of oxygen that can be transported from the lungs to the working muscles in heavy or exhausting exercise (see *oxygen transport*). Thus maximal work capacity refers to the specific work load that elicits VO_2 max.

maximal heart rate   The highest heart rate that an individual can attain; predicted by the formula (220 minus age) equals maximal heart rate.

metabolism   The chemical processes catalyzed by specialized proteins (enzymes) that are carried out in every cell.

minerals   The crystalline chemical elements or compounds essential for cellular metabolism; essential in every tissue and fluid in the body.

mitochondria   The components of a cell, located where energy is generated, that carry out metabolism.

ml. O_2/min./kg.   Milliliters of oxygen consumed per minute, divided by body mass in kilograms; the measure of maximal oxygen consumption during exercise. Since it is expressed in terms of body size, it allows subjects of varying sizes to be compared relatively.

muscle fiber   The basic structural unit of muscle; the muscle cell.

muscular endurance   The ability of a muscle to perform repeated contractions against a resistance.

muscular–endurance exercises   Repetitive, submaximal muscular contractions, measured by the time to fatigue and performed by the major muscle groups of the body.

myocardial infarction   An interruption of blood supply to the myocardium (heart muscle) resulting in permanent tissue damage.

Newton (N) Unit of measurement of force.

nutrition The study of food and the six essential nutrients: water, vitamins, minerals, proteins, carbohydrates, and fats.

obesity An excessive percentage of fat in the body mass: more than 25 percent for males, more than 30 percent for females.

overload principle A greater-than-normal load placed on muscle or muscle groups in order to increase their strength.

oxygen The gas that constitutes 20.93 percent of air; an essential component of metabolism and must be transported to the cells of the body.

oxygen transport (Vo_2 consumption) in exercise The delivery of oxygen by the lungs, heart, blood, and vascular system to the working muscles, where large quantities of it are needed for the aerobic production of energy.

parturition The process of birth.

physiology The study of the systems and processes of the body. Exercise physiology deals in the study of these systems and processes during exercise.

plasma The fluid portion (approximately 60 percent) of the blood.

power The rate of doing work that requires large amounts of anaerobic energy; moving a load through a distance over time.

protein A complex molecule made up of many amino acids; forms the basic structure of the cell.

pulmonary function The relative functional health of the pulmonary system (the lungs).

red blood cells The cells that transport oxygen; hemaglobin is located inside each red blood cell. Most of the hematocrit is red blood cells.

repetitions The consecutive number of contractions (usually 5 to 10) performed during one exercise set; a term applied specifically to strength exercises in which implements (free weights or machines) are used. A set should be repeated 3 times, with suitable rest periods in between.

respiration The process of gas exchange both in the lungs and in the cells.

sarcolemma The cell membrane of muscle fiber.

sarcoplasm The protoplasm of muscle cells.

saturated fats Foods obtained primarily from animal sources, such as meat and dairy products.

slow–twitch muscle fiber The type of muscle fiber used during repetitive endurance activities, such as running and swimming.

step test   A submaximal exercise that measures the heart-rate recovery after stepping on and off a bench for three minutes.

strain-mechanical   The deformation within a structure while it is being loaded.

strength   The maximal capacity of a muscle or muscle group to exert force against a resistance.

stress-mechanical   The load per unit area that develops in response to a force that is applied from without.

stretching   The movement of a body part through the full range of motion in order to maintain or improve its flexibility.

stroke volume   The volume of blood squeezed out from the left ventricle during a heart beat by contraction of the ventricular musculature.

subcutaneous fat   Fat deposited in the adipose tissue immediately under the skin's surface; constitutes approximately 80 percent of the body's stored fat. The amount of fat deposited varies with the individual, the location on the body, and gender.

sugar   An edible form of carbohydrate used as an energy source in the body.

systolic blood pressure   The greatest pressure exerted by the blood against the walls of the arteries; usually measured on the upper arm just above the elbow, at the level of the heart.

tendon   Connective tissue that attaches muscle to the periosteum of bone.

training   Repeated exercises that are highly sports-specific; training should never be confused with exercise prescription.

triglyceride   Body fat that is stored economically in the adipose tissues in the form of 3 attached fatty acids.

unsaturated fats   Foods obtained primarily from vegetable sources, such as edible oils and nuts.

vascular system   The tubular blood-conduction network of the body, composed of arteries, veins, and capillaries.

vein   The portion of the vascular system that carries blood from the tissues back to the heart.

ventilation   The movement of air into and then out of the lungs; measured in liters per minute.

ventricles   The chambers in the heart that pump blood to the lungs (right ventricle) and throughout the body (left ventricle).

vitamins Organic substances that perform important regulatory functions in the body.

Vo₂ Oxygen consumption.

warm-up The first phase of any exercise prescription. The warm-up prepares the body for the activity to follow.

Appendices

Appendix A: Anatomy Diagrams and Muscle Action Tables

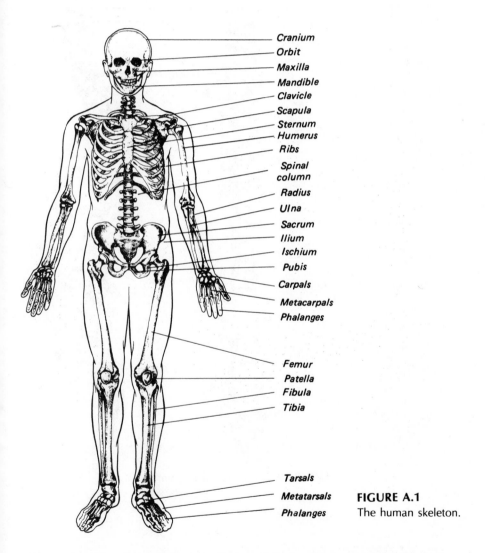

- Cranium
- Orbit
- Maxilla
- Mandible
- Clavicle
- Scapula
- Sternum
- Humerus
- Ribs
- Spinal column
- Radius
- Ulna
- Sacrum
- Ilium
- Ischium
- Pubis
- Carpals
- Metacarpals
- Phalanges
- Femur
- Patella
- Fibula
- Tibia
- Tarsals
- Metatarsals
- Phalanges

FIGURE A.1
The human skeleton.

Figures A.1–A.9 from James G. Hay and J. Gavin Reid, *The Anatomical and Mechanical Bases of Human Motion,* © 1982, pp. 385–390. Reprinted by permission of Prentice-Hall, Inc., Englewood Cliffs, N.J.

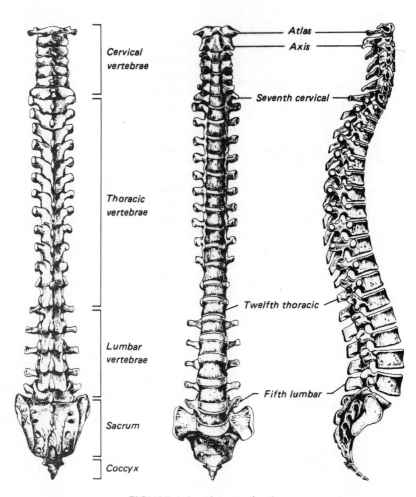

FIGURE A.2 The spinal column.

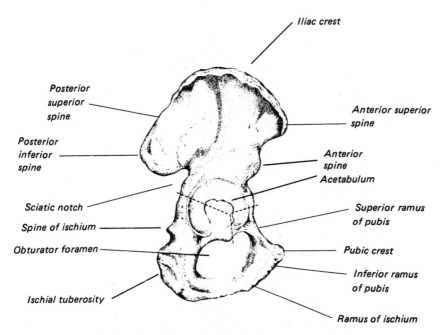

FIGURE A.3   Lateral view of the right side of the pelvis.

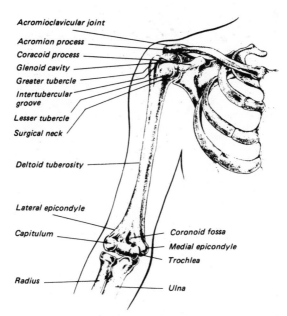

FIGURE A.4   The shoulder girdle, shoulder joint, and humerus.

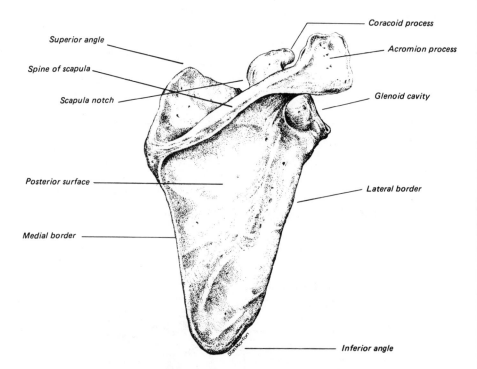

FIGURE A.5   The scapula.

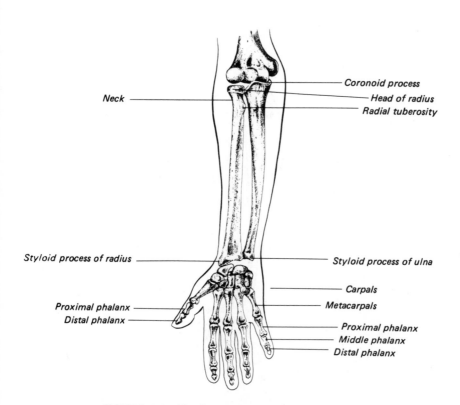

Neck

Styloid process of radius

Proximal phalanx
Distal phalanx

Coronoid process
Head of radius
Radial tuberosity

Styloid process of ulna

Carpals
Metacarpals

Proximal phalanx
Middle phalanx
Distal phalanx

FIGURE A.6   The forearm and hand (anterior view).

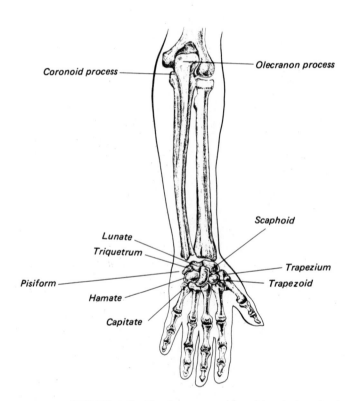

FIGURE A.7 The forearm and hand (posterior view).

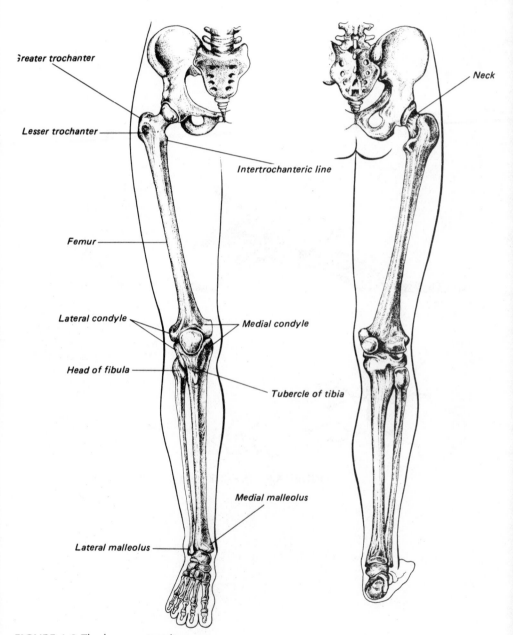

FIGURE A.8 The lower extremity.

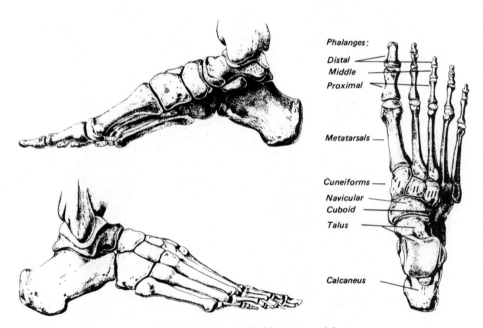

FIGURE A.9   The ankle joint and foot.

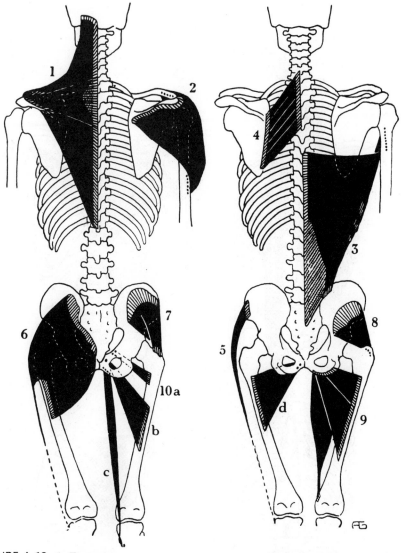

FIGURE A.10
1. Trapezius
2. Deltoid
3. Latissimus dorsi
4. Rhomboids
5. Tensor fasciae latae
6. Gluteus maximus
7. Gluteus medius

8. Gluteus minimus
9. Adductor magnus
10. a) Pectineus
    b) Adductor longus
    c) Adductor gracilis
    d) Adductor brevis

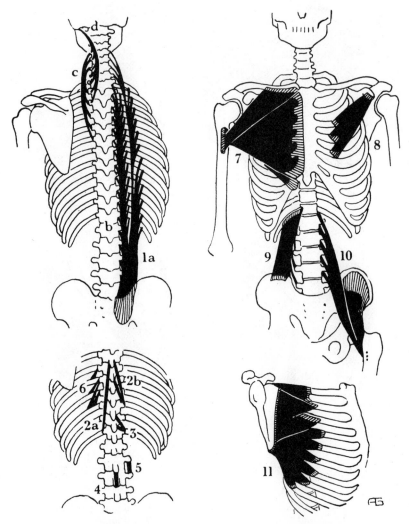

FIGURE A.11

1. Sacrospinalis
   a) Iliocostalis
   b,c,d) Longissimus dorsi
2. a) Semispinalis
   b) Multifidus
3. Rotators
4. Interspinalis

5. Intertransversarii
6. Levator costarum
7. Pectoralis major
8. Pectoralis minor
9. Quadratus lumborum
10. Iliopsoas
11. Serratus anterior

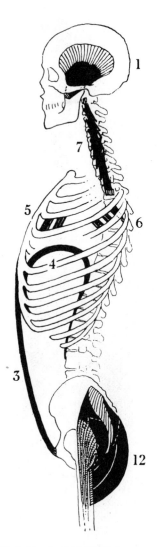
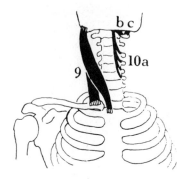
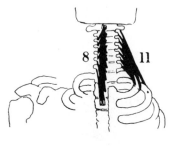
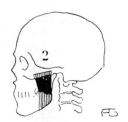

FIGURE A.12   1. Temporalis
2. Masseter
3. Rectus abdominis
4. Diaphragm
5. External intercostals
6. Internal intercostals

7,8. Longus colli
9. Sternocleidomastoid
10. a) Longus capitis
    b,c) Rectus capitus
11. Scalenius
12. Gluteus maximus

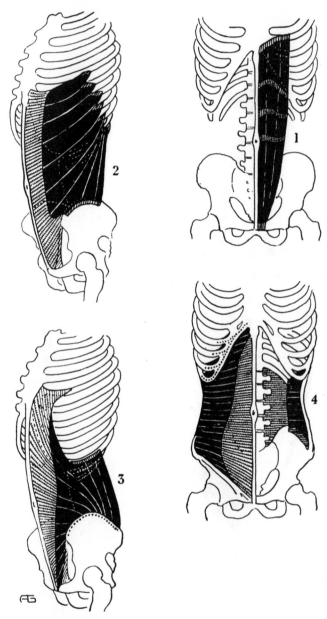

FIGURE A.13   1. Rectus abdominis
2. External oblique
3. Internal oblique
4. Transversus abdominis

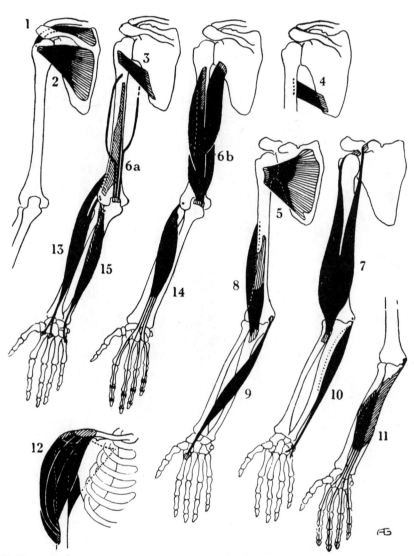

FIGURE A.14

1. Supraspinatus
2. Infraspinatus
3. Teres minor
4. Teres major
5. Subscapularis
6. Triceps brachii
7. Biceps brachii
8. Brachialis
9. Flexor carpi radialis
10. Flexor carpi ulnaris
11. Flexor digitorum sublimis and profundus
12. Deltoid
13. Extensor carpi radialis longus and brevis
14. Extensor digitorum communis
15. Extensor carpi ulnaris

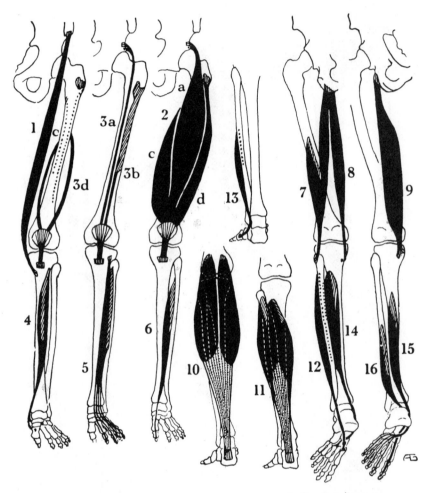

FIGURE A.15
1. Sartorius
2. Quadriceps femoris
3. a) Rectus femoris
   b) Vastus intermedius
   c) Vastus medialis
   d) Vastus lateralis
4. Tibialis anterior
5. Extensor digitorum longus
6. Extensor hallucis longus
7. Biceps femoris

8. Semitendinosus
9. Semimembranosus
10. Gastroenemius
11. Soleus
12. Peroneus longus
13. Peroneus brevis
14. Tibialis posterior
15. Flexor digitorum longus
16. Flexor hallucis longus

TABLE A.1 Muscles Acting on the Neck

MUSCLE	LOCATION	ORIGIN	INSERTION	ACTION
Longissimus capitis	Posterior-lateral neck	Articular processes of lower 3 or 4 cervical vertebrae and transverse processes of upper 4 or 5 thoracic vertebrae	Temporal bone (mastoid process)	Extends neck. Singly: bends neck to side and rotates head toward contracting side.
Semispinalis capitis	Posterior neck	Transverse processes of seventh cervical and superior 6 or 7 thoracic vertebrae	Occipital bone	Extends neck. Singly: rotates head to same side.
Splenius capitis	Posterior neck	Inferior half ligamentum nuchae, spine of seventh cervical and superior 3 or 4 thoracic vertebrae	Occipital bone, temporal bone (mastoid process)	Extends neck. Singly: rotates head to same side.
Sternocleidomastoid	Lateral neck	Sternum (manubrium), clavicle	Temporal bone (mastoid process)	Flexes neck. Singly: rotates head toward opposite side of contracting muscle.

Tables A.1–A.11 from James G. Hay and J. Gavin Reid, *The Anatomical and Mechanical Bases of Human Motion*, © 1982, pp. 397–407. Reprinted by permission of Prentice-Hall, Inc., Englewood Cliffs, N.J.

TABLE A.2 Muscles of the Abdominal Wall (Anterior Trunk)

MUSCLE	LOCATION	ORIGIN	INSERTION	ACTION
External oblique	Anterior abdominal (superficial)	Anterior inferior aspect of lower 8 ribs	Iliac crest, linea alba, pubic tubercle	Compresses, supports abdominal viscera, flexion, and rotation. Singly: lateral bending of spine.
Internal oblique	Anterior and lateral abdominal deep to external oblique	Lateral portion of inguinal ligament, iliac crest, and thoracolumbar fascia	Cartilage of lower 3 ribs, linea alba	Compresses abdomen; assists in forced breathing (expiration). Singly: assists in lateral trunk bending; assists in flexion of spine.
Rectus abdominis	Anterior midline of abdomen (superficial)	Symphysics pubis and crest of pubis	Sternum (xiphoid process) and cartilage of fifth, sixth, and seventh ribs	Flexes vertebral column; compresses abdominal viscera; assists in breathing.
Transversus abdominis	Abdominal deep layer	Inguinal ligament, iliac crest, cartilages of lower 6 ribs, and lumbar fascia	Xiphoid process, linea alba, and pubis	Compresses abdomen; assists in forced expiration.

TABLE A.3 Muscles of the Trunk (Posterior)

MUSCLE	LOCATION	ORIGIN	INSERTION	ACTION
Erector spinae (sacrospinalis); includes iliocostalis, longissimus, spinalis	Length of back (sacrum to skull)	Iliac crest, sacrum, ribs, transverse and spinous processes of most lumbar and thoracic vertebrae	Ribs; transverse processes of second to sixth cervical, all thoracic, and the upper lumbar vertebrae; spines of upper thoracic vertebrae; temporal and occipital bones	Extends, bends laterally, and rotates vertebral column.
Quadratus lumborum	Between iliac crest and lower rib	Iliac crest (posterior), iliolumbar ligament	Lower rib, transverse processes of upper four lumbar vertebrae	Extends lumbar spine. Singly: bends spinal column laterally.

TABLE A.4 Muscles Used in Respiration*

MUSCLE	LOCATION	ORIGIN	INSERTION	ACTION
Diaphragm	Between abdominal and thoracic cavities	Xiphoid process, costal cartilages of lower 6 ribs, and lumbocostal arches	Central tendon	Contraction; increases thoracic cavity; aids in respiration.
External intercostals (eleven pairs)	Between ribs (superficial)	Inferior border of rib above	Superior border of rib below	Elevates ribs in inspiration.
Internal intercostals	Between ribs (deep)	Superior border of rib below	Inferior border of rib above	Draws adjacent ribs together during forced expiration.

*Note Table A.2.

TABLE A.5 Muscles Acting on the Shoulder Girdle

MUSCLE	LOCATION	ORIGIN	INSERTION	ACTION
Levator scapulae	Neck (posterior)	First 4 cervical vertebrae	Medial border of scapula from the spine to the superior angle	Elevates scapula.
Pectoralis minor	Chest (deep to pectoralis major)	Ribs (third to fifth)	Scapula (coracoid process)	Depresses scapula; pulls shoulder forward.
Rhomboid major	Deep upper back	Spinous processes (second to fifth thoracic vertebrae)	Medial border of scapula (spine to inferior angle)	Adducts and rotates scapula.
Rhomboid minor	Deep upper back, superior and superficial to major	Ligamentum nuchae (lower part), seventh cervical and first thoracic vertebrae	Scapula spine (root)	Adducts scapula.
Serratus anterior	Lateral thorax	Upper 8 or 9 ribs	Medial border of scapula	Abducts scapula.
Trapezius	Upper back and neck (superficial)	Occipital protuberance, ligamentum nuchae, spine of seventh cervical and all thoracic vertebrae	Clavicle, spine of scapula, and acromion process	Adducts and rotates scapula; elevates and depresses scapula; extends neck. Singly: bends neck laterally.

TABLE A.6 Muscles Acting on the Upper Arm (Shoulder Joint)

MUSCLE	LOCATION	ORIGIN	INSERTION	ACTION
Coracobrachialis	Upper arm (medial)	Scapula (coracoid process)	Humerus (middle of medial surface)	Flexes and adducts.
Deltoid	Anterior, lateral, and posterior upper surface of humerus	Clavicle, scapula (acromion and spine)	Deltoid tuberosity of humerus	Abducts arms. Parts: flexes, extends, and rotates.
Infraspinatus	Posterior surface of scapula below spine	Scapula (infraspinous fossa)	Greater tuberosity of humerus	Rotates humerus laterally.
Latissimus dorsi	Lower back (superficial)	Vertebrae spines (thoracic sixth through twelfth lumbar and sacral), lumbosacral fascia, crest of ilium, muscular slips from lower 3 or 4 ribs	Humerus (bicipital groove)	Adducts, extends, and medially rotates humerus.
Pectoralis major	Chest			
Clavicular pectoralis		Clavicle (medial half)	Humerus (lateral lip of bicipital groove)	Flexes and medially rotates humerus.
Sternocostal pectoralis		Sternum and costal cartilages of true ribs	Humerus (lateral lip of bicipital groove)	Extends, adducts, and medially rotates humerus.
Supraspinatus	Posterior surface of scapula above spine	Scapula (supraspinous fossa)	Humerus (greater tuberosity)	Adducts humerus (assists).
Teres major	Inferior angle of scapula to humerus	Scapula (dorsal surface, inferior angle)	Humerus (bicipital groove)	Adducts, extends, and medially rotates humerus.
Teres minor	Immediately superior to teres major	Scapula (dorsal surface of lateral border)	Humerus (greater tuberosity)	Adducts and rotates humerus laterally.

TABLE A.7 Muscles Acting on the Forearm

MUSCLE	LOCATION	ORIGIN	INSERTION	ACTION
Biceps brachii	Upper arm (anterior and superficial)	Short head: scapula (coracoid process); long head: scapula (supraglenoid tuberosity)	Radial tuberosity, deep fascia of forearm	Flexes and supinates forearm.
Brachialis	Upper arm (lower two thirds, anterior and deep)	Humerus (lower two-thirds of anterior surface)	Ulna (coronoid process and tuberosity)	Flexes forearm.
Brachioradialis	Lateral forearm	Humerus (superior two-thirds of lateral supracondylar ridge)	Radius (styloid process)	Flexes forearm.
Pronator quadratus	Anterior forearm (distal end and deep)	Ulna (distal portion on shaft, anterior surface)	Radius (distal fourth, lateral border)	Pronates forearm.
Pronator teres	Anterior upper forearm	Humerus (medial epicondyle), ulna (coronoid process)	Radius (middle portion, lateral side)	Pronates and flexes forearm.
Supinator	Anterior upper forearm (deep to pronator teres and brachioradialis)	Humerus (lateral epicondyle), radius (ridge below radial notch)	Radius (proximal third lateral and anterior surface)	Supinates forearm.
Triceps brachii	Posterior humerus	Long head: scapula (infra-glenoid tuberosity); medial head: humerus (lower surface); lateral head (above radial groove)	Ulna (olecranon process)	Extends forearm.
Anconeus	Posterior elbow	Lateral epicondyle of humerus	Olecranon process and ulna	Extends elbow; pronates forearm.

TABLE A.8 Muscles That Move the Wrist and Hand

MUSCLE	LOCATION	ORIGIN	INSERTION	ACTION
Extensor carpi radialis longus	Posterior forearm	Humerus (lateral supracondylar ridge)	Second metacarpal (base)	Extends wrist; abducts hand.
Extensor carpi radialis brevis	Posterior forearm	Humerus (lateral epicondyle)	Third metacarpal (base)	Extends wrist; abducts hand.
Extensor carpi ulnaris	Posterior forearm	Humerus (lateral epicondyle), ulna (proximal half of shaft)	Fifth metacarpal (base)	Extends wrist; adducts hand.
Extensor digitorum	Posterior forearm	Humerus (lateral epicondyle)	Fingers (middle and distal phalanges)	Extends phalanges.
Extensor indicis	Posterior forearm (distal end)	Ulna (distal surface)	Index finger (proximal phalanx)	Extends proximal phalanx of index finger.
Flexor carpi radialis	Anterior forearm (superficial)	Humerus (medial epicondyle)	Second and third metacarpals (base)	Flexes wrist; abducts hands; assists elbow flexion.
Flexor carpi ulnaris	Anterior forearm (superficial)	Humerus (medial epicondyle), ulna (proximal two-thirds)	Pisiform, hamate, base of fifth metacarpal	Flexes wrist; adducts hands; assists in elbow flexion.
Flexor digitorum profundus	Anterior forearm (deep)	Ulna (medial and anterior surface), deep fascia	Fingers (base of distal phalanges)	Flexes distal phalanges.
Flexor digitorum superficialis	Anterior forearm (medium)	Humerus (medial epicondyle), ulna (coronoid process), radius (oblique line)	Fingers (base of second phalanx)	Flexes second phalanx of fingers; flexes hand; assists in elbow flexion.
Palmaris longus	Anterior forearm	Humerus (medial epicondyle)	Palmar aponeurosis	Flexes wrist.

TABLE A.9 Muscles Acting on the Thigh (Hip Joint)

MUSCLE	LOCATION	ORIGIN	INSERTION	ACTION
Abductor group				
Magnus	Medial thigh	Rami of ischium and pubis, ischial tuberosity	Femur (greater trochanter to linea aspera), linea aspera, supracondylar line, adductor tubercle	Adducts, flexes, extends, and rotates thigh.
Longus	Medial thigh	Pubis (crest and symphysis)	Femur (linea aspera, middle third)	Adducts, flexes, and rotates thigh.
Brevis	Medial thigh	Pubis (inferior ramus)	Femur (linea aspera)	Adducts, flexes, and rotates thigh.
Gluteal group				
Maximus	Buttocks (superficial)	Ilium (posterior gluteal line), sacrum and coccyx (posterior surface), sacrotuberous ligament	Femur (greater tuberosity), iliotibial tract	Extends, abducts, and laterally rotates thigh; extends lower trunk.
Medius	Buttocks (intermediate)	Ilium (outer surface and crest)	Femur (greater trochanter)	Abducts and medially rotates thigh.

Muscle	Location	Origin	Insertion	Action
Minimus	Buttocks (deep)	Ilium (inferior to medius)	Femur (anterior surface of greater trochanter)	Abducts and medially rotates thigh.
Gracilis	Medial thigh	Symphysis pubis (inferior aspect)	Tibia (proximal end medial surface)	Adducts thigh; flexes and medially rotates leg.
Iliopsoas	Posterior wall of pelvic cavity	Vertebrae (transverse processes and bodies of twelfth thoracic and all lumbar), iliac fossa	Femur (lesser trochanter)	Flexes thigh; flexes lumbar region on thigh.
Pectineus	Medial thigh	Pubis (pectineal line and fascia)	Femur (pectineal line)	Flexes and adducts thigh.
Piriformis	Posterior pelvis (deep)	Sacrum (anterior surface), sacrotuberous ligament	Femur (greater trochanter)	Abducts and laterally rotates thigh.
Rectus femoris	anterior thigh (superficial)	Ilium (anterior inferior iliac spine), groove on acetabulum	Tibia (patella tendon)	(Flexes thigh; extends leg.
Sartorius	Anterior and medial thigh (superficial)	Ilium (anterior superior iliac spine)	Tibia (proximal end, medial surface)	Flexes thigh and rotates it laterally; flexes leg.
Tensor fasciae latae	Lateral hip and proximal thigh	Ilium (anterior part of crest)	Iliotibial tract of fasciae lata	Flexes, abducts, and medially rotates thigh; tenses fasciae lata.
Hamstring group	Posterior thigh	(see Table A.10)		

TABLE A.10 Muscles Acting on the Leg (Knee Joint)

MUSCLE	LOCATION	ORIGIN	INSERTION	ACTION
Hamstring group				
Biceps femoris	Posterior thigh (superficial)	Ischium (tuberosity and sacrotuberous ligament), femur (linea aspera)	Fibula (head), tibia (lateral condyle)	Flexes lg and extends thigh (rotates leg laterally when knee is flexed).
Semitendinosus	Posterior thigh (medial)	Ischium (tuberosity)	Tibia (proximal end, medial surface)	Flexes leg and extends thigh (rotates leg medially when knee is flexed).
Semimembranosus	Posterior thigh	Ischium (tuberosity)	Tibia (medial condyle)	Flexes leg and extends thigh (rotates leg medially when knee is flexed).
Quadriceps femoris group				
Rectus femoris	Anterior thigh (superficial)	Ilium (anterior inferior iliac spine), groove on acetabulum	Patella (patella ligament to tibial tubercle)	Extends leg and flexes thigh.
Vastus lateralis	Lateral thigh	Femur (linea aspera and greater trochanter)	Lateral border of patellar ligament (to tibial tubercle)	Extends leg.
Vastus medialis	Medial thigh	Femur (upper portion of medial aspect of shaft)	Medial border of patellar ligament to tibial tubercle	Extends leg.
Vastus intermedius	Anterior thigh (deep)	Femur (anterior surface)	Patellar ligament to tibial tubercle	Extends leg.
Gracilis	Medial thigh (superficial)	Symphysis pubis	Tibia (proximal end, medial surface)	Flexes and medially rotates leg; adducts thigh.
Sartorius	Anterior and medial thigh (superficial)	Ilium (anterior superior iliac spine)	Tibia (proximal end, medial surface)	Flexes leg; flexes thigh and rotates it laterally.
Popliteus	Posterior knee	Femur (lateral condyle and popliteal ligament)	Tibia (superior to popliteal line, posterior aspect)	Rotates femur laterally on tibia

TABLE A.11 Muscles That Move the Foot

MUSCLE	LOCATION	ORIGIN	INSERTION	ACTION
Extensor digitorum longus	Anteriolateral leg	Tibia (lateral condyle), fibula (anterior surface), interosseous membrane	Four lateral toes (second and third phalanges)	Extends phalanges; dorsiflexes foot.
Extensor hallucis longus	Anterior fibula	Fibula (middle half of shaft), interosseous membrane	Great toe (base of distal phalanx)	Extends great toe; aids dorsiflexion of foot.
Flexor digitorum longus	Posterior tibia	Tibia (posterior shaft)	Distal phalanges of lateral four toes	Flexes distal phalanges; aids in plantar flexion.
Flexor hallucis longus	Posterior fibula	Fibula (distal two-thirds of shaft), interosseous membrane	Distal phalanx of great toe	Flexes great toe; aids in plantar flexion.
Gastrocnemius	Calf of leg (superficial)	Lateral head: femur (lateral condyle); Medial head: femur (medial condyle)	Calcaneus (by calcaneal tendon)	Plantar-flexes the foot; flexes the leg.

(continued)

TABLE A.11 Muscles That Move the Foot (*continued*)

MUSCLE	LOCATION	ORIGIN	INSERTION	ACTION
Peroneus brevis	Lateral leg	Fibula (distal two-thirds of lateral surface of shaft)	Fifth metatarsal (base on lateral side)	Plantar-flexes; everts foot.
Peroneus longus	Lateral leg	Tibia (lateral condyle), fibula (head and proximal two-thirds of shaft)	Medial cuneiform and base of first metatarsal	Plantar-flexes; everts foot.
Peroneus tertius	Anterior fibula (distal end)	Fibula (distal anterior surface)	Fifth metatarsal (base)	Dorsiflexes and everts foot.
Soleus	Calf of leg (deep to gastrocnemius)	Tibia (middle third), fibula (head and proximal third of shaft)	Calcaneus (by calcaneal tendon)	Plantar-flexes foot.
Tibialis anterior	Anterior fibula	Tibia (lateral condyle, proximal two-thirds of shaft)	Medial cuneiform and metatarsal (base of first)	Dorsiflexes and inverts foot.
Tibialis posterior	Posterior leg (deep to soleus)	Tibia and fibula (shaft) interosseous membrane	Navicular, cuneiforms, second, third, and fourth metatarsals (base) and cuboid	Plantar-flexes and inverts foot.

Appendix B: The Metric System

The metric system, known also as the Système International d'Unités (S.I.), is used throughout much of the world in science, engineering, education, and everyday living. Table B.1 lists the measures used in this text and gives their abbreviation symbols. Table B.2 presents a simple means of converting back and forth between equivalent metric and American units of measure.

TABLE B.1   Basic Units and Symbols of S.I.

MEASUREMENT	NAME OF UNIT	SYMBOL
length	meter	m
mass	kilogram	kg
speed	meters per second	m/s
force	Newton	N

TABLE B.2 Conversion Factors (Rounded Off to Nearest One-Thousandth)

LENGTH

METERS	YARDS	FEET	INCHES
1	1.094	3.281	39.370
0.914	1	3	36
0.305	0.333	1	12
0.025	0.028	0.083	1
0.315	0.344	1.033	12.396

KILOMETERS	MILES
1	0.621
1.609	1

Meters to yards: Yards to meters:
multiply by 1.0946   multiply by 0.914

Kilometers to miles: Miles to kilometers:
multiply by 0.6214   multiply by 1.609

MASS

KILOGRAMS	POUNDS (avoirdupois)
1	2.205
0.494	1

Kilograms to pounds: Pounds to kilograms:
multiply by 2.205   multiply by 0.494

SPEED

Meters per second	Kilometers per hour	Feet per second	Miles per hour
1	3.6	3.281	2.237
0.278	1	0.911	0.621
0.305	1.097	1	0.682
0.447	1.609	1.467	1
0.515	1.853	1.689	1.152
0.514	1.852	1.688	1.151

Meters per second to miles per hour:
multiply by 2.237

Miles per hour to meters per second:
multiply by 0.447

FORCE

NEWTONS	POUNDS
1	0.225
4.448	1

Newtons to pounds: Pounds to Newtons:
multiply by 0.2248   multiply by 4.448

Appendix C: Quantity and Quality
of Exercise
Recommended for Fitness

Increasing numbers of persons are becoming involved in endurance training activities and thus, the need for guidelines for exercise prescription is apparent.

Based on the existing evidence concerning exercise prescription for healthy adults and the need for guidelines, the American College of Sports Medicine makes the following recommendations for the quantity and quality of training for developing and maintaining cardiorespiratory fitness and body composition in the healthy adult:

1. Frequency of training: 3 to 5 days per week.
2. Intensity of training: 60% to 90% of maximum heart rate reserve or, 50% to 85% of maximum oxygen uptake ($\dot{V}O_2$ max).
3. Duration of training: 15 to 60 minutes of continuous aerobic activity. Duration is dependent on the intensity of the activity, thus lower intensity activity should be conducted over a longer period of time. Because of the importance of the "total fitness" effect and the fact that it is more readily attained in longer duration programs, and because of the potential hazards and compliance problems associated with high intensity activity, lower to moderate intensity activity of longer duration is recommended for the non-athletic adult.
4. Mode of activity: Any activity that uses large muscle groups, that can be maintained continuously, and is rhythmical and aerobic in nature, e.g. running-jogging, walking-hiking, swimming, skating, bicycling, rowing, cross-country skiing, rope skipping, and various endurance game activities.

Position statement by the American College of Sports Medicine on "The Recommended Quantity and Quality of Exercise for Developing and Maintaining Fitness in Healthy Adults." From the *Journal of Medicine and Science in Sports*, vol. 10, no. 3, 1978. Reprinted by permission of the American College of Sports Medicine.

Rationale and Research Background

The questions "How much exercise is enough and what type of exercise is best for developing and maintaining fitness?" are frequently asked. It is recognized that the term *physical fitness* is composed of a wide variety of variables included in the broad categories of cardiovascular-respiratory fitness, physique and structure, motor function, and many histochemical and biochemical factors. It is also recognized that the adaptative response to training is complex and includes peripheral, central, structural, and functional factors. Although many such variables and their adaptative response to training have been documented, the lack of sufficient in-depth and comparative data relative to frequency, intensity, and duration of training make them inadequate to use as comparative models. Thus, in respect to the above questions, fitness will be limited to changes in $\dot{V}O_2$ max, total body mass, fat weight (FW), and lean body weight (LBW) factors.

Exercise prescription is based upon the frequency, intensity, and duration of training, the mode of activity (aerobic in nature, e.g. listed under No. 4 above), and the initial level of fitness. In evaluating these factors, the following observations have been derived from studies conducted with endurance training programs.

1. Improvement in $\dot{V}O_2$ max is directly related to frequency (2,23,32, 58,59,65,77,79), intensity (2,10,13,26,33, 37,42,56,77), and duration (3,14,29,49,56, 77,86) of training. Depending upon the quantity and quality of training, improvement in $\dot{V}O_2$ max ranges from 5% to 25% (4,13,27,31,35,36,43,45,52,53, 62,71,77,78, 82,86). Although changes in $\dot{V}O_2$ max greater than 25% have been shown, they are usually associated with large total body mass and FW loss, or a low initial level of fitness. Also, as a result of leg fatigue or a lack of motivation, persons with low initial fitness may have spuriously low initial $\dot{V}O_2$ max values.

2. The amount of improvement in $\dot{V}O_2$ max tends to plateau when frequency of training is increased above 3 days per week (23,62,65). For the non-athlete, there is not enough information available at this time to speculate on the value of added improvement found in programs that are conducted more than 5 days per week. Participation of less than two days per week does not show an adequate change in $\dot{V}O_2$ max (24,56,62).

3. Total body mass and FW are generally reduced with endurance training programs (67), while LBW remains constant (62,67,87) or increases slightly (54). Programs that are conducted at least 3 days per week (58,59,61,62,87), of at least 20 minutes duration (48,62,87) and of sufficient intensity and duration to expend approximately 300 kilocalories (Kcal) per exercise session are suggested as a threshold level for total body mass and FW loss (12,29,62,67). An expenditure of 200 Kcal per session has also been shown to be useful in weight reduction if the exercise frequency is at least 4 days per week (80). Programs with less participation generally show little or no change in body composition (19,25,42,62,67,84,85,87). Significant increases in $\dot{V}O_2$ max have been shown with 10 to 15 minutes of high intensity training (34,49,56,62,77,78). Thus, if total body mass and FW reduction is not a consideration, then short duration, high intensity programs may be recommended for healthy, low risk (cardiovascular disease) persons.

4. The minimal threshold level for improvement in $\dot{V}O_2$ max is approximately 60% of the maximum heart rate reserve (50% of $\dot{V}O_2$ max) (33,37). Maximum heart rate reserve represents the percent difference between resting and maximum heart rate, added to the resting heart rate. The technique, as described by Karvonen, Kentala, and Mustala (37), was validated by Davis and Convertino (14), and represents a heart rate of approximately 130 to 135 beats/minute for young persons. As a result of the aging curve for maximum heart rate, the absolute heart rate value (threshold level) is inversely related to age, and can be as low as 110 to 120 beats/minute for older persons. Initial level of fitness is another important consideration in prescribing exercise (10,40,46,75,77). The person

with a low fitness level can get a significant training effect with a sustained training heart rate as low as 110 to 120 beats/minute, while persons of higher fitness levels need a higher threshold of stimulation (26).

5. Intensity and duration of training are interrelated, with the total amount of work accomplished being an important factor in improvement in fitness (2,7,12, 40,61,62,76,78). Although more comprehensive inquiry is necessary, present evidence suggests that when exercise is performed above the minimal threshold of intensity, the total amount of work accomplished is the important factor in fitness development (2,7,12,61,62,76,79) and maintenance (68). That is, improvement will be similar for activities performed at a lower intensity–longer duration compared to higher intensity–shorter duration if the total energy costs of the activities are equal.

If frequency, intensity, and duration of training are similar (total Kcal expenditure), the training result appears to be independent of the mode of aerobic activity (56,60,62,64). Therefore, a variety of endurance activities, e.g. listed above, may be used to derive the same training effect.

6. In order to maintain the training effect, exercise must be continued on a regular basis (2,6,11,21,44,73,74). A significant reduction in working capacity occurs after two weeks of detraining (73) with participants returning to near pretraining levels of fitness after 10 weeks (21) to 8 months of detraining (44). Fifty percent reduction on improvement of cardiorespiratory fitness has been shown after 4 to 12 weeks of detraining (21, 41,73). More investigation is necessary to evaluate the rate of increase and decrease of fitness with varying training loads and reduction in training in relation to level of fitness, age, and length of time in training. Also, more information is needed to better identify the minimal level of work necessary to maintain fitness.

7. Endurance activities that require running and jumping generally cause significantly more debilitating injuries to beginning exercisers than other non-weight bearing activities (42,55,69). One study showed that beginning joggers had increased foot, leg, and knee injuries when training was performed more than 3 days per week and longer than 30 minutes duration per exercise session (69). Thus, caution should be taken when recommending the type of activity and exercise prescription for the beginning exerciser. Also, the increase of orthopedic injuries as related to overuse (marathon training) with chronic jogger-runners is apparent. Thus, there is a need for more inquiry into the effect that different types of activities and the quantity and quality of training have on short-term and long-term participation.

8. Most of the information concerning training described in this position statement has been conducted on men. The lack of information on women is apparent, but the available evidence indicates that women tend to adapt to endurance training in the same manner as men (8,22,89).

9. Age in itself does not appear to be a deterrent to endurance training. Although some earlier studies showed a lower training effect with middle-aged or elderly participants (4,17,34,83,86), more recent study shows the relative change in $\dot{V}O_2$ max to be similar to younger age groups (3,52,66,75,86). Although more investigation is necessary concerning the rate of improvement in $\dot{V}O_2$ max with age, at present it appears that elderly participants need longer periods of time to adapt to training (17,66). Earlier studies showing moderate to no improvement in $\dot{V}O_2$ max were conducted over a short time-span (4) or exercise was conducted at a moderate to low Kcal expenditure (17), thus making the interpretation of the results difficult.

Although $\dot{V}O_2$ max decreases with age, and total body mass and FW increase with age, evidence suggests that this trend can be altered with endurance training (9,12,38,39,62). Also, 5 to 10 year follow-up studies where participants continued their training at a similar level showed maintenance of fitness (39,70). A study of older competitive runners showed decreases in $\dot{V}O_2$ max from the fourth to seventh decade of life, but also showed reductions in their training load (63). More inquiry into the relationship of long-term training (quantity and quality) for both competitors and non-competitors and physiological function with increasing age, is necessary before more definitive statements can be made.

10. An activity such as weight training should not be considered as a means of training for developing $\dot{V}_{O_2}$ max, but has significant value for increasing muscular strength and endurance, and LBW (16,24,47,49,88). Recent studies evaluating circuit weight training (weight training conducted almost continuously with moderate weights, using 10 to 15 repetitions per exercise session with 15 to 30 seconds rest between bouts of activity) showed little to no improvements in working capacity and $\dot{V}_{O_2}$ max (1,24,90).

Despite an abundance of information available concerning the training of the human organism, the lack of standardization of testing protocols and procedures, methodology in relation to training procedures and experimental design, and a preciseness in the documentation and reporting of the quantity and quality of training prescribed, make interpretation difficult (62,67). Interpretation and comparison of results are also dependent on the initial level of fitness (18,74–76,81), length of time of the training experiment (20,57,58,61,62), and specificity of the testing and training (64). For example, data from training studies using subjects with varied levels of $\dot{V}_{O_2}$ max, total body mass, and FW have found changes to occur in relation to their initial values (5,15,48,50,51), i.e., the lower the initial $\dot{V}_{O_2}$ max the larger the percent of improvement found, and the higher the FW the greater the reduction. Also, data evaluating trainability with age, comparison of the different magnitudes and quantities of effort, and comparison of the trainability of men and women may have been influenced by the initial fitness levels.

In view of the fact that improvement in the fitness variables discussed in this position statement continues over many months of training (12,38,39,62), it is reasonable to believe that short-term studies conducted over a few weeks have certain limitations. Middle-aged sedentary and older participants may take several weeks to adapt to the initial rigors of training, and thus need a longer adaptation period

to get the full benefit from a program. How long a training experiment should be conducted is difficult to determine, but 15 to 20 weeks may be a good minimum standard. For example, two investigations conducted with middle-aged men who jogged either 2 or 4 days per week found both groups to improve in $\dot{V}_{O_2}$ max. Mid-test results of the 16 and 20 week programs showed no difference between groups, while subsequent final testing found the 4 day per week group to improve significantly more (58,59). In a similar study with young college men, no differences in $\dot{V}_{O_2}$ max were found among groups after 7 and 13 weeks of interval training (20). These latter findings and those of other investigators point to the limitations in interpreting results from investigations conducted over a short time-span (62,67).

In summary, frequency, intensity and duration of training have been found to be effective stimuli for producing a training effect. In general, the lower the stimuli, the lower the training effect (2,12,13, 27,35,46,77,78,90), and the greater the stimuli, the greater the effect (2,12, 13,27,58,77,78). It has also been shown that endurance training less than 2 days per week, less than 50% of maximum oxygen uptake, and less than 10 minutes per day is inadequate for developing and maintaining fitness for healthy adults.

REFERENCES

1. Allen, T. E., R. J. Byrd and D. P. Smith. Hemodynamic consequences of circuit weight training. *Res. Q.* 43:299–306, 1976.

2. American College of Sports Medicine. *Guidelines for Graded Exercise Testing and Exercise Prescription*. Philadelphia: Lea and Febiger, 1976.

3. Barry, A. J., J. W. Daly, E. D. R. Pruett, J. R. Steinmetz, H. F. Page, N. C. Birkhead and K. Rodahl. The effects of physical conditioning on older individuals. I. Work capacity, circulatory-respiratory function, and work electrocardiogram. *J. Gerontol.* 21: 182–191, 1966.

4. Bensetad, A. M. Trainability of old men. *Acta. Med. Scandinav.* 178:321–327, 1965.

5. Boileau, R. A., E. R. Buskirk, D. H. Horstman, J. Mendez and W. C. Nicholas. Body composition changes in obese and lean men during physical conditioning. *Med. Sci. Sports* 3:183–189, 1971.

6. Brynteson, P. and W. E. Sinning. The effects of training frequencies on the retension of cardiovascular fitness. *Med. Sci. Sports* 5:29–33, 1973.

7. Burke, E. J. and B. D. Franks. Changes in $\dot{V}O_2$ max resulting from bicycle training at different intensities holding total mechanical work constant. *Res. Q.* 46:31–37, 1975.

8. Burke, E. J. Physiological effects of similar training programs in males and females. *Res. Q.* 48:510–517, 1977.

9. Carter, J. E. L. and W. H. Phillips. Structural changes in exercising middle-aged males during a 2-year period. *J. Appl. Physiol.* 27:787–794, 1969.

10. Crews, T. R. and J. A. Roberts. Effects of interaction of frequency and intensity of training. *Res. Q.* 47:48–55, 1976.

11. Cureton, T. K. and E. E. Phillips. Physical fitness changes in middle-aged men attributable to equal eight-week periods of training, non-training and retraining. *J. Sports Med. Phys. Fitness* 4:1–7, 1964.

12. Cureton, T. K. *The Physiological Effects of Exercise Programs upon Adults.* Springfield: Charles C. Thomas, 1969.

13. Davies, C. T. M. and A. V. Knibbs. The training stimulus, the effects of intensity, duration and frequency of effort on maximum aerobic power output. *Int. Z. Angew. Physiol.* 29:299–305, 1971.

14. Davis, J. A. and V. A. Convertino. A comparison of heart rate methods for predicting endurance training intensity. *Med. Sci. Sports* 7:295–298, 1975.

15. Dempsey, J. A. Anthropometrical observations on obese and non-obese young men undergoing a program of vigorous physical exercise. *Res. Q.* 35:275–287, 1964.

16. Delorme, T. L. Restoration of muscle power by heavy resistance exercise. *J. Bone and Joint Surgery* 27:645–667, 1945.

17. DeVries, H. A. Physiological effects of an exercise training regimen upon men aged 52 to 88. *J. Gerontol.* 24:325–336, 1970.

18. Ekblom, B., P. O. Åstrand, B. Saltin, J. Sternberg and B. Wallstrom. Effect of training on circulatory response to exercise. *J. Appl. Physiol.* 24:518–528, 1968.

19. Flint, M. M., B. L. Drinkwater and S. M. Horvath. Effects of training on women's response to submaximal exercise. *Med. Sci. Sports* 6:89–94, 1974.

20. Fox, E. L., R. L. Bartels, C. E. Billings, R. O'Brien, R. Bason and D. K. Mathews. Frequency and duration of interval training programs and changes in aerobic power. *J. Appl. Physiol.* 38:481–484, 1975.

21. Fringer, M. N. and A. G. Stull. Changes in cardiorespiratory parameters during periods of training and detraining in young female adults. *Med. Sci. Sports* 6:20–25, 1974.

22. Getchell, L. H. and J. C. Moore. Physical training: comparative responses of middle-aged adults. *Arch. Phys. Med. Rehab.* 56:250–254, 1975.

23. Gettman, L. R., M. L. Pollock, J. L. Durstine, A. Ward, J. Ayres and A. C. Linnerud. Physiological responses of men to 1, 3, and 5 day per week training programs. *Res. Q.* 47:638–646, 1976.

24. Gettman, L. R., J. Ayres, M. L. Pollock, J. L. Durstine and W. Grantham. Physiological effects of circuit strength training and jogging on adult men. *Arch. Phys. Med. Rehab.*, in press.

25. Girandola, R. N. Body composition changes in women: Effects of high and low exercise intensity. *Arch Phys. Med. Rehab.* 57:297–300, 1976.

26. Gledhill, N. and R. B. Eynon. The intensity of training. In: A. W. Taylor and M. L. Howell (editors). *Training Scientific Basis and Application.* Springfield: Charles C. Thomas, pp. 97–102, 1972.

27. Golding, L. Effects of physical training upon total serum cholesterol levels. *Res. Q.* 32:499–505, 1961.

28. Goode, R. C., A. Virgin, T. T. Romet, P. Crawford, J. Duffin, T. Pallandi and Z. Woch. Effects of a short period of physical activity in adolescent boys and girls. *Canad. J. Appl. Sports Sci.* 1:241–250, 1976.

29. Gwinup, G. Effect of exercise alone on the weight of obese women. *Arch. Int. Med.* 135:676–680, 1975.

30. Hanson, J. S., B. S. Tabakin, A. M. Levy and W. Nedde. Long-term physical training

and cardiovascular dynamics in middle-aged men. *Circ.* 38:783–799, 1968.

31. Hartley, L. H., G. Grimby, A. Kilbom, N. J. Nilsson, I. Asthand, J. Bjure, B. Ekblom and B. Saltin. Physical training in sedentary middle-aged and older men. *Scand. J. Clin. Lab. Invest.* 24:335–344, 1969.

32. Hill, J. S. The effects of frequency of exercise on cardiorespiratory fitness of adult men. M. S. Thesis, Univ. of Western Ontario, London, 1969.

33. Hollmann, W. and H. Venrath. Experimentelle Untersuchungen zur Bedeutung eines Trainings unterhalb und oberhalb der Dauerbeltz Stungsgrenze. In: Korbs (editor). *Carl Diem Festschrift.* W. u. a. Frankfurt/Wein, 1962.

34. Hollman, W. Changes in the capacity for maximal and continuous effort in relation to age. *Int. Res. Sport Phys. Ed.,* (E. Jokl and E. Simon, editors). Springfield: Charles C. Thomas, 1964.

35. Huibregtse, W. H., H. H. Hartley, L. R. Jones, W. D. Doolittle and T. L. Criblez. Improvement of aerobic work capacity following non-strenuous exercise. *Arch. Env. Health,* 27:12–15, 1973.

36. Ismail, A. H., D. Corrigan and D. F. McLeod. Effect of an eight-month exercise program on selected physiological, biochemical, and audiological variables in adult men. *Brit. J. Sports Med.* 7:230–240, 1973.

37. Karvonen, M., K. Kentala and O. Mustala. The effects of training heart rate: A longitudinal study. *Ann. Med. Exptl. Biol. Fenn.* 35:307–315, 1957.

38. Kasch, F. W., W. H. Phillips, J. E. L. Carter and J. L. Boyer. Cardiovascular changes in middle-aged men during two years of training. *J. Appl. Physiol. 314:53–57, 1972.*

39. Kasch, F. W. and J. P. Wallace. Physiological variables during 10 years of endurance exercise. *Med. Sci. Sports* 8:5–8, 1976.

40. Kearney, J. T., A. G. Stull, J. L. Ewing and J. W. Strein. Cardiorespiratory responses of sedentary college women as a function of training intensity. *J. Appl. Physiol.* 41:822–825, 1976.

41. Kendrick, Z. B., M. L. Pollock, T. N. Hickman and H. S. Miller. Effects of training and detraining on cardiovascular efficiency. *Amer. Corr. Ther. J.* 25:79–83, 1971.

42. Kilbom, A., L. Hartley, B. Saltin, J. Bjure,

G. Grimby and I. Åstrand. Physical training in sedentary middle-aged and older men. *Scand. J. Clin. Lab. Invest.* 24:315–322, 1969.

43. Knehr, C. A., D. B. Dill and W. Neufeld. Training and its effect on man at rest and at work. *Amer. J. Physiol.* 136:148–156, 1942.

44. Knuttgen, H. G., L. O. Nordesjo, B. Ollander and B. Saltin. Physical conditioning through interval training with young male adults. *Med. Sci. Sports* 5:220–226, 1973.

45. Mann, G. V., L. H. Garrett, A. Farhi, H. Murray, T. F. Billings, F. Shute and S. E. Schwarten. Exercise to prevent coronary heart disease. *Amer. J. Med.* 46:12–27, 1969.

46. Marigold, E. A. The effect of training at predetermined heart rate levels for sedentary college women. *Med. Sci. Sports* 6:14–19, 1974.

47. Mayhew, J. L. and P. M. Gross. Body composition changes in young women with high resistance weight training. *Res. Q.* 45:433–439, 1974.

48. Milesis, C. A., M. L. Pollock, M. D. Bah, J. J. Ayres, A. Ward and A. C. Linnerud. Effects of different durations of training on cardiorespiratory function, body composition and serum lipids. *Res. Q.* 47:716–725, 1976.

49. Misner, J. E., R. A. Boileau, B. H. Massey and J. H. Mayhew. Alterations in body composition of adult men during selected physical training programs. *J. Amer. Geriatr. Soc.* 22:33–38, 1974.

50. Moody, D. I., J. Kollias and E. R. Buskirk. The effect of a moderate exercise program on body weight and shinfold thickness in overweight college women. *Med. Sci. Sports* 1:75–80, 1969.

51. Moody, D. L., J. H. Wilmore, R. N. Girandola and J. P. Royce. The effects of a jogging program on the body composition of normal and obese high school girls. *Med. Sci. Sports* 4:210–213, 1972.

52. Myrhe, L., S. Robinson, A. Brown and F. Pyke. Paper presented to the American College of Sports Medicine, Albuquerque, New Mexico, 1970.

53. Naughton, J. and F. Nagle. Peak oxygen intake during physical fitness program for middle-aged men. *JAMA* 191:899–901, 1965.

54. O'Hara, W., C. Allen and R. J. Shephard. Loss of body weight and fat during exercise in a cold chamber. *Europ. J. Appl. Physiol.* 37:205–218, 1977.

55. Oja, P., P. Teraslinna, T. Partaner and R. Karava. Feasibility of an 18 months' physical training program for middle-aged men and its effect on physical fitness. *Am. J. Public Health* 64:459–465, 1975.

56. Olree, H. D., B. Corbin, J. Penrod and C. Smith. Methods of achieving and maintaining physical fitness for prolonged space flight. Final Progress Rep. to NASA, Grant No. NGR-04-002-004, 1969.

57. Oscai, L. B., T. Williams and B. Hertig. Effects of exercise on blood volume. *J. Appl. Physiol.* 24:622–624, 1968.

58. Pollock, M. L., T. K. Cureton and L. Greninger. Effects of frequency of training on working capacity, cardiovascular function, and body composition of adult men. *Med. Sci. Sports* 1:70–74, 1969.

59. Pollock, M. L., J. Tiffany, L. Gettman, R. Janeway and H. Lofland. Effects of frequency of training on serum lipids, cardiovascular function, and body composition. In: *Exercise and fitness* (B. D. Franks, editor), Chicago: Athletic Institute, 1969, pp. 161–178.

60. Pollock, M. L., H. Miller, R. Janeway, A. C. Linnerud, B. Robertson and R. Valentino. Effects of walking on body composition and cardiovascular function of middle-aged men. *J. Appl. Physiol.* 30:126–130, 1971.

61. Pollock, M. L., J. Broida, Z. Kendrick, H. S. Miller, R. Janeway and A. C. Linnerud. Effects of training two days per week at different intensities on middle-aged men. *Med. Sci. Sports* 4:192–197, 1972.

62. Pollock, M. L. The quantification of endurance training programs. *Exercise and Sport Sciences Reviews,* (J. Wilmore, editor). New York: Academic Press, pp. 155–188, 1973.

63. Pollock, M. L., H. S. Miller, Jr. and J. Wilmore. Physiological characteristics of champion American track athletes 40 to 70 years of age. *J. Gerontol.* 29:645–649, 1974.

64. Pollock, M. L., J. Dimmick, H. S. Miller, Z. Kendrick and A. C. Linnerud. Effects of mode of training on cardiovascular function and body composition of middle-aged men. *Med. Sci. Sports* 7:139–145, 1975.

65. Pollock, M. L., H. S. Miller, A. C. Linnerud and K. H. Cooper. Frequency of training as a determinant for improvement in cardiovascular function and body composition of middle-aged men. *Arch. Phys. Med. Rehab.* 56:141–145, 1975.

66. Pollock, M. L., G. A. Dawson, H. S. Miller, Jr., A. Ward, D. Cooper, W. Headly, A. C. Linnerud and M. M. Nomeir. Physiologic response of men 49 to 65 years of age to endurance training. *J. Amer. Geriatr. Soc.* 24:97–104, 1976.

67. Pollock, M. L. and A. Jackson. Body Composition: Measurement and changes resulting from physical training. Proceedings National College Physical Education Association for Men and Women, pp. 125–137, January, 1977.

68. Pollock, M. L., J. Ayres and A. Ward. Cardiorespiratory fitness: Response to differing intensities and durations of training. *Arch. Phys. Med. Rehab.* 58:467–473, 1977.

69. Pollock, M. L., L. R. Gettman, C. A. Milesis, M. D. Bah, J. L. Durstine and R. B. Johnson. Effects of frequency and duration of training on attrition and incidence of injury. *Med. Sci. Sports* 9:31–36, 1977.

70. Pollock, M. L., H. S. Miller and P. M. Ribisl. Body composition and cardiorespiratory fitness in former athletes. *Phys. Sports Med.,* In press, 1978.

71. Ribisl, P. M. Effects of training upon the maximal oxygen uptake of middle-aged men. *Int. Z. Angew. Physiol.* 26:272–278, 1969.

72. Robinson, S. and P. M. Harmon. Lactic acid mechanism and certain properties of blood in relation to training. *Amer. J. Physiol.* 132:757–769, 1941.

73. Roskamm, H. Optimum patterns of exercise for healthy adults. *Canad. Med. Ass. J.* 96:895–899, 1967.

74. Saltin, B., G. Blomqvist, J. Mitchell, R. L., Johnson, K. Wildenthal and C. B. Chapman. Response to exercise after bed rest and after training. *Circ.* 37 and 38. Supp. 7, 1–78, 1968.

75. Saltin, B., L. Hartley, A. Kilbom and I. Åstrand. Physical training in sedentary middle-aged and older men. *Scand. J. Clin. Lab. Invest.* 24:323–334, 1969.

76. Sharkey, B. J. Intensity and duration of training and the development of cardiores-

piratory endurance. *Med. Sci. Sports* 2:197–202, 1970.

77. Shephard, R. J. Intensity, duration, and frequency of exercise as determinants of the response to a training regime. *Int. Z. Angew. Physiol.* 26:272–278, 1969.

78. Shephard, R. J. Future research on the quantifying of endurance training. *J. Human Ergology.* 3:163–181, 1975.

79. Sidney, K. H., R. B. Eynon and D. A. Cunningham. Effect of frequency of training of exercise upon physical working performance and selected variables representative of cardiorespiratory fitness. In: *Training Scientific Basis and Application* (A. W. Taylor editor) Springfield: Charles C. Thomas, pp. 144–188, 1972.

80. Sidney, K. H., R. J. Shephard and J. Harrison. Endurance training and body composition of the elderly. *Amer. J. Clin. Nutr.* 30:326–333, 1977.

81. Siegel, W., G. Blomqvist and J. H. Mitchell. Effects of a quantitated physical training program on middle-aged sedentary males. *Circ.* 41:19, 1970.

82. Skinner, J., J. Holloszy and T. Cureton. Effects of a program of endurance exercise on physical work capacity and anthropometric measurements of fifteen middle-aged men. *Amer. J. Cardiol.* 14:747–752, 1964.

83. Skinner, J. The cardiovascular system with aging and exercise. In: Brunner, D. and E. Jokl (editors). *Physical Activity and Aging* Baltimore: University Park Press, 1970, pp. 100–108.

84. Smith, D. P. and F. W. Stransky. The effect of training and detraining on the body composition and cardiovascular response of young women to exercise. *J. Sports Med.* 16:112–120, 1976.

85. Terjung, R. L., K. M. Baldwin, J. Cooksey, B. Samson and R. A. Sutter. Cardiovascular adaptation to twelve minutes of mild daily exercise in middle-aged sedentary men. *J. Amer. Geriatr. Soc.* 21:164–168, 1973.

86. Wilmore, J. H., J. Royce, R. N. Girandola, F. I. Katch and V. I. Katch. Physiological alterations resulting from a 10-week jogging program. *Med. Sci. Sports* 2(1):7–14, 1970.

87. Wilmore, J. H., J. Royce, R. N. Girandola, F. I. Katch and V. I. Katch. Body composition changes with a 10-week jogging program. *Med. Sci. Sports* 2:113–117, 1970.

88. Wilmore, J. H. Alterations in strength, body composition, and anthropometric measurements consequent to a 10-week weight training program. *Med. Sci. Sports* 6:133–138, 1974.

89. Wilmore, J. Inferiority of female athletes: Myth or reality. *J. Sports Med.* 3:1–6, 1974.

90. Wilmore, J., R. B. Parr, P. A. Vodak, T. J. Barstow, T. V. Pipes, A. Ward and P. Leslie. Strength, endurance BMR, and body composition changes with circuit weight training. (Abstract) *Med. Sci. Sports* 8:58–60, 1976.

Index